I0510598

My Dominican Experience

A Medical School Journey

A MEMOIR

By

Frank E. Robinson, MD

Copyright © 2017 by Frank E. Robinson, MD

All rights reserved.

ISBN-13: 978-1546814078

Cover Art includes the Dominican Republic flag and abstractly depicts the assistance I received from many generous people who I encountered during medical school.

DEDICATIONS

I would like to dedicate this memoir, My Dominican Experience, to my Mom, Marian Miller Hankerson, whose strong spiritual foundation, tireless nurturing and constant encouragement provided me with the strong foundation I would rely upon during my arduous pursuit to become a physician. This personal tome is also dedicated to my Dad, Frank Robinson, who instilled in me the solid principles of fearlessness, discipline and being true to who you are.

To both of them, I am forever humbly grateful !

FRANK E. ROBINSON, MD

ACKNOWLEDGMENTS

My Dominican Experience was the outgrowth from a conversation I had with a friend in Greensboro, NC many years ago, by the name of Dr.John Raye. Over coffee I told Dr. Raye, incidentally of my journey overseas as a medical student. He was quite astounded with the very fact that I'd actually gone to a foreign country to study medicine. He took copious notes as we conversed and said, "Son, you have the making of a helluva story …. You have to tell it, this will be an inspiration for many !"

I actually began writing my autobiography a couple of years ago and the Dominican experience was included in one of the chapters. One day, I recalled Dr. Raye's words and thought, the Dominican experience is a book within itself. I began putting pen to paper and expanded the chapter and thus began the book, My Dominican Experience. The writing of this memoir wouldn't have been accomplished or completed without the aid, assistance and support of many. I want to first thank my lovely wife and life partner, Karen Collins Robinson for her patience and continued love, both during the actual Dominican experience, as well as her time in reading and rereading the manuscript to ensure all details were true and accurate.

Of course, none of the memoir would have gotten to any stage of completion without the many long hours put in by my brother Gilbert (Gil) Robinson. No words can express my gratitude to him for his efforts in reading my initial writings, making corrections, suggesting better sentence structure and in providing general good advice. He had the patience, and knowledge to put my words into a form and structure that would convey the meaning I was attempting to relay to the reader.

I want to also thank my typist Ms. Bernice Easley for typing the manuscript on a very tight time schedule. My editor, Ms. Vicki Bleus, was a blessing. She was there at the right time and was able to proof and edit my document and get it ready for formatting. Last but not least, I want to thank Ms. Sabrina Scott for her tireless efforts over several months in patiently guiding me through this, my first publication. She coordinated the process to ensure I followed all steps necessary, including formatting, cover design, copyrighting and publisher selection all in an effort to produce a quality book.

FRANK E. ROBINSON, MD

FAVORITE QUOTES

"If you have a brain, use it ! It's all you need to overcome any problem!"
- Dr. Ben Carson in "Take The Risk"

"The Ladder of Success is never crowded at the top."
- Florence Griffith Joyner

"I did the best I could, with what I had."
- Justice Thurgood Marshall

"The man who views the world at fifty the same as he did at twenty has wasted thirty years of his life."
- Muhammad Ali

"It is quite easy to shout slogans, to sign manifestos, but it is quite a different matter to build, manage, command, spend days and nights seeking the solution of problems."
- Patrice Lumumba

"Show me someone content with mediocrity and I'll show you someone destined for failure."
- Dr. Johnetta Cole

"Agitate, Agitate, Agitate !!"
- Frederick Douglass

FRANK E. ROBINSON, MD

INTRODUCTION

This is a short story, a memoir of a black man's journey from the streets of Newark, NJ in the 1970's as he navigated the landmines of the US educational system. Dr. Frank Robinson delves into a vital and important portion of his pursuit to attain one of the highest and acclaimed educational degrees in this country, the Doctor of Medicine. In this memoir, the reader is given a snapshot from his autobiography, entitled "This is as Good As It Gets", during a most uncertain and tumultuous time in his life … getting into medical school.

One might say many persons have gone to medical school. This is certainly true, but few have done it the way Dr. Frank Robinson did it! What is most fascinating, interesting, and detailed in this memoir is the route Dr. Robinson took in his journey. The memoir covers the time Dr. Robinson spent in medical school, first in the Dominican Republic for two years and then state-side at Rutgers Medical School in Camden, NJ. Yes, Dr. Robinson actually went to, lived in, and studied during his first two medical school years in Santo Domingo, Dominican Republic, that small Caribbean island, formerly known as Hispaniola which it shares with Haiti. As you will read, what is interesting are the dilemmas and choices he confronted. The decisions he had to make and the risks he took were remarkable, considering where he started.

As a teenager, his desire to become a doctor never waned. Once he had set his sights on medicine, nothing else came even close to holding his interest. Of course, this "poor" 14 year-old kid from the streets of Newark, NJ had no idea what he was getting into. On television and in the movies, doctors and lawyers had already completed medical and law school and were in full fledge practice mode. Hollywood and idealism at their best. There was no mention of all the years of sacrifice, study, and long hours it took for them to make complicated diagnoses, perform complex surgeries, or argue cases successfully before a judge.

Perhaps it was fortunate he was not aware of all the pitfalls and challenges that were ahead. Such forewarning just may have served as a deterrent to the young man. Sometimes wide-eyed innocence, ignorance, and youthful exuberance can work in one's favor. Finally, none of my brother's accomplishments would have been possible if it had not been for the inspiration, encouragement, and love of his wife, Karen Lorraine Robinson. Not only have they worked as a team, she was unyielding in her support and continually had her husband's back as a registered nurse during all the years of schooling, frequent moves, and job changes. I might add, she also managed the household in his absence and cared for their young and growing children.

The life and career of Dr. Frank Robinson can serve as a reminder to any young person, particularly young African Americans, that despite where you start in life, be it the streets of Newark, NJ or anywhere else in this country, you can achieve what you desire in life. You must find your passion and pursue it with every ounce of your God given ability. Never ever give up! One of Dr. Robinson's favorite quotes is, "If at least one person has done it, then I can do it!"

Gilbert A. Robinson

Chapter One

On a cool fall afternoon in the late 1970's in East Orange, NJ
where we lived while I was pursuing my Bachelor's Degree at
Rutgers University in Newark, NJ, I returned to our apartment. As
usual, it had been a long day. As I opened the day's mail, I noticed
the usual thin envelope. Even without opening it I knew its
contents: another medical school rejection. I had applied to a
number of medical schools, mostly in the northeast, in the fall as is
the custom for those seeking admission to medical school. Up to
this point, I had received rejection after rejection. As you might
imagine, it became more difficult mentally and emotionally to
maintain my focus and direction in the face of this seemingly grim
situation. Would I ever get a big envelope signaling admission?
Would I ever be able to tell friends and call family to say that I had
been accepted to med school?

As I received the last of the thin rejection letters, I regained my composure and began to examine and evaluate my options. My wife, Karen, and I talked about the situation and the future that awaited me and us as a family. What were my options? What else could I do with the Bachelor's Degree in Zoology and Physiology that I would receive shortly in May 1979. I had worked part-time as a lab tech at area companies in New Jersey and was not really interested in pursuing this as a career. I pondered and pondered my options and wondered what else was there. I read many career and health occupational manuals in the Dana Library at Rutgers. At this point, we had been married for only five or six months and Karen was now pregnant with our first child, Kamilah who was due in November 1979.

The stress was mounting to do something. I found it! I had heard about Physician's Assistants (PAs) for a number of years. I began to read more about the profession and what PAs did. I liked what I read. I called the school in Brooklyn, NY which had a program at Long Island University. I did not know any PAs personally, but it sounded like something very close to what I wanted to do in medicine, short of being an MD. I received the application by mail, completed it, and went for the interview. I was accepted and began matriculation in the summer of 1979.

I was able to complete the requisite courses in the PA program and graduated in August 1981. I took my first job as a PA at the Methadone Clinic for Beth Israel Hospital in Harlem, NY. This clinic was located at 125th Street and Park Avenue near the subway train which was elevated at the time. I was accustomed to working in Harlem since I had done so while selling clothes on the Harlem streets in the early 70's. I had fond memories and learned a lot about the streets during that time. Now, however, I was a health professional and the lens through which I saw the world, and Harlem in particular, was quite different. I was older and my focus now was quite different. In addition, our second daughter, Aquilah was born in September about two weeks before I started the Methadone Clinic job so things were certainly moving fast and we needed the extra income. I had acquired a couple of student loans during my time at Rutgers and also at Long Island University.

I remained at the Harlem job for three or four months. I learned a lot about drug abuse while there and made a few friends in the clinic. The drug culture is a culture all of its own. The communication I needed for the patrons at the Methadone Clinic was one I had to acquire. I had to be streetwise and trust no one. There was also a strong Caribbean influence in Brooklyn and in Harlem. I would say I spent more time around Jamaicans and Haitians over this period of time than black Americans. I learned a lot about the Caribbean culture and its food.

After leaving the Harlem clinic, my good friend from PA school, Frank Ognelodgh (Frank O), referred me to the Medical Director at

New York Prison Health, Dr. Wallace Rooney. He and I became good friends and he was very helpful in later years as there were times when I needed part-time work. Dr. Rooney always looked out for me. Also, I worked at a pediatric clinic in Brooklyn on Gates Avenue which was owned and operated by a pediatrician, the late Dr. Darryl Morton.

Later, I settled into a clinic on Greene Street near downtown Brooklyn by the name of HIRE which stood for Health Is Right for Everyone. It was at HIRE where I met and worked with a great group of doctors that would ultimately give me the inspiration and courage to look into a method and means to accomplish my dream: that ultimate dream of becoming a medical doctor. I cannot thank those doctors enough for the push and inspiration that propelled me to go for it all. They were special in the sense that they had all been born in Caribbean islands and studied medicine there; not as US citizens, but as native Caribbean islanders. Over the years since becoming a physician, it was not American physicians, for the most part, who were essential in my becoming a physician. It was foreign trained doctors working in the United States who served as that impetus for me to continue on.

Chapter 2

Prior to working at the HIRE medical facility in 1980, I had covered the pediatric clinic at Mid-Brooklyn Health Care where the administrator was Mr. Waldabah Stewart. He was a shrewd businessman from the Caribbean who operated a tight ship. He was a very good employer who understood the health care structure and system of New York City and in particular, Brooklyn.

My medical director at Mid-Brooklyn was an internist named Dr. Miguel Cerone whose home was in the Dominican Republic. He was a very quiet, shy doctor who missed being away from his home in Santo Domingo. He did not like the harsh cold winters of New York but was continuing to work in the United States to earn a higher income to assist in his retirement as well as to financially assist his daughter Caroline through medical school at the main university in the Dominican Republic. Dr. Cerone and I became close friends and many years later I had an opportunity to visit him at his beautiful, spacious home in Santo Domingo and meet his lovely wife and daughter.

The majority of my PA work time, however, was spent at HIRE. The Executive Director was Mr. Curtis Evans and the Medical Director was Dr. Jean Etienne, a Haitian internist. The clinic was located in a three-story building owned by Dr. Josephine English who was an OB-GYN physician by training. She was famous in that she had delivered the children of Malcolm X (aka El-Hajj Malik el-Shabazz). Dr. English was an older physician who did not look her age and was very sharp intellectually and knew her stuff, in business and in medicine. She was an exceptional gynecologist.

I had a great time at HIRE and made a lot of friends who I would ultimately need and reference in my quest to become a doctor. I worked closely with PA Vernon Williams, my closet friend in Brooklyn besides Frank O. Vernon was much older than me and pushed the heck out of me. He would not allow me to settle for anything less than the best that I could become. Vernon always emphasized that average was not good enough. I also worked with and learned a lot from Pediatrician Dr. Wilfred Florvil, as well as Dr. Monsanto and Dr. Roger Tarter, all of whom had varying personalities. They were a great group to work with in addition to a general surgeon who came in once a week by the name of Dr. Mozhanzadeh who was from Iran.

I also worked with some wonderful ladies: Linda Askew, a registered nurse, Carmen Rosa, a Puerto Rican nurse's aide and a clerical staff member consisting of Delphina Anderson and Audrey (who last name escapes me). In addition, there was Mr. Curtis who was a virtual jack of all trades and the Center's van driver. He and Vernon were always at each other, mentally challenging one another.

Chapter 3

My experience in Brooklyn was my first entry to the multiculturalism of blacks, other than African Americans, and to this day I value that exposure and experience. It opened my eyes and expanded my vision of life and was the beginning of a new awareness of the world and of things other than what I had grown up in and around Newark. I think we often miss opportunities for growth in life because we are not open to new ideas, beliefs, and customs.

I have learned that people tend to navigate in a narrow, constricted zone of comfort and have a fear of challenging or questioning their own long held-beliefs or paradigms. I believe knowledge is power and a tool and if sought after, utilized, and put into action can take you far beyond your wildest imagination. Fear is a natural human emotion that if embraced and held too strongly will stymie even the most courageous individual. Zig Ziglar, the late motivator

9

speaker, described FEAR with the acrostic:

F(False) E(Expectation) A(Appearing) R(Real)

I remember a conversation I had with Dr. Etienne one day regarding medical school and my thoughts on wanting to attend one outside of the United States. He was from Haiti and had graduated from medical school there. He told me that many Americans were being accepted into medical schools in the Caribbean and Mexico and were practicing in the United States after completing their coursework and graduating. Dr. Etienne strongly encouraged me to apply without hesitation or reservation.

This valuable and surprising piece of information I received from Dr. Etienne and others piqued my interest and ignited my intense immediate research into these off-shore schools. Bear in mind, this was before the days of the internet and the world wide web so all research was done through the library and via cold calls and handwritten letters, many letters. I spoke to everyone I could about the possibility of going to medical school overseas and discovered that many schools had cropped up over the preceding five years in Mexico and the Caribbean catering to Americans who were unable to achieve admission to mainland US medical schools.

Prior to this, Americans for decades had gone to medical schools in Italy, Brussels, France, Switzerland, and Canada. I further discovered that most of those students studying in the Islands and Mexico were Caucasians! To my amazement, very few blacks, to my knowledge knew of, or if they did, didn't have the courage to even entertain the idea of studying medicine overseas.

As with any investigation or pursuit of this type (and life in general), several obstacles and potential roadblocks began to appear that placed an immediate cloud over my aspirations. Number one, most if not all schools required tuition payments in cash. There were no loan programs, grants, or scholarships. Secondly, most of the school's curriculums were taught in Spanish or the language of that particular country. For example, in Italy (Italian) or Montreal Canada (French), etc. ... but, several medical schools, due to the high number of Americans applying, were starting to offer curriculums taught in English. As you can imagine, medical school taught in English is a daunting task in and of itself and the thought of possibly having to deal with classes taught in a foreign language was not a challenge I looked forward to confronting with great enthusiasm. But I was determined to do what I had to do to get the job done.

Another issue I personally had to overcome was I had a family consisting of a wife and two young children, ages one and two at home! We had moved into a two-bedroom apartment at 133 Cleveland Street in Orange, NJ shortly after Aquilah (the youngest child) was born in 1981 so that the kids would have a separate bedroom. Up to that point, we all slept in the one-bedroom apartment on Glenwood Avenue in East Orange. Karen at this time was working at the University of Medicine and Dentistry on Bergen Street in Newark as a Clinical Nurse Specialist and thus we had a decent income to cover our basic expenses. In addition, she had purchased a 1978 Chevy Impala a couple of years prior so we had a reliable mode of transportation for her and our children. I continued to work at HIRE as well as several fill-in odd part-time PA jobs in Brooklyn while driving several different used cars with "may pop" tires! I worked everywhere I could find work Mondays through Saturdays and if there was work on Sundays, I did that also. If it was legal and not unethical I did it.

As one can imagine, Karen and I had to resolve these issues one at a time and see how this adventure could be accomplished. There was no doubt in my mind that it would be done. I just needed to figure out the how! I had only been working full-time for about six months and did not have much in savings. I was already working six to seven days a week as it was, going to multiple clinics and doing other odd jobs. I was young, hungry, and definitely not lazy. My philosophy then as it is now was that no one owed me anything and if I am to be successful and achieve anything in life it was totally up to me with no excuses. I strongly believe God (The Creator) helps only those who help themselves! In this situation, I needed to sit down at the drawing board and map out a strategy after getting some numbers from the various schools and figure out how to do it financially.

Once I had compiled information on several schools, I applied only to those schools that taught exclusively in English. What's interesting is that I did not even think at that time about airfare or room and board. I figured I would get those "little" details taken care of later. I applied to several schools and was accepted at Cifas, Cetec, and Universidad Mundial-Dominicana (World University) aka Mundial.

As part of my due diligence, I bought a ticket and flew to the Dominican Republic in early 1982 to visit and see if the schools were real and not some kind of scam. After arriving in the Dominican Republic, I rented a car and visited the campuses of Cifas, Cetec, and Mundial over a couple of days and spoke with students and faculty. Of all the schools, Mundial was the smallest and least known. I stayed in the Naco region of Santo Domingo at the Hotel Naco. The weather was beautiful and the people were friendly and helpful. Of course, I had my Spanish dictionary with me and the people tended to be very open to individuals who at least attempted to speak their native language.

For some reason, I was most impressed with Mundial though there were a lot more Americans at Cifas and Cetec. Something about Mundial was more personable and less Americanized. In any event, my mind was made up to attend Mundial and whether it was

Divine Providence or not, over the years it turned out to be a wise choice. While economic and political scandals ensnared many other schools, Mundial was one of the few schools that avoided these issues and eventual closure. I attributed this to its small, unassuming size and its dedication to education, not just making money.

My acceptance letter from Mundial was dated January 22, 1982 and classes were scheduled to begin May 17, 1982. For a number of reasons, there was no way I could meet this deadline. I telephoned Dr. Carlos Lastra, Dean of Admissions and Committee Chairman, to request a transfer of my start date and the school agreed to move it to September 13, 1982. A $500 deposit was required as well as half of the first semester's tuition which was $2,000. I did my usual hustling (working like hell) and came up with the $1,500 (not a small sum in those days) and mailed it in to reserve my spot for the fall term. It was only after this that I told Karen I was going. I wanted a definite, not a probable or a maybe, before I broke the news to her. This wasn't an easy time, there was a lot of stress and a gazillion unknowns. They say ignorance is bliss and that certainly applied in my case. I was determined to go to med school come hell or high water. It didn't really matter how I was going to do it, but I knew I had to do it. I was one driven and on-fire brother!

Chapter 4

Needless to say, there was some consternation on Karen's part as well as some "silent" reservations mostly from Uncle John (Karen's uncle). Interestingly, Aunt Carrie (Karen's aunt) was more in favor than the others. I think her thought was, this guy (me) is working very hard towards his goal of studying medicine and she did not see that in a lot of black men. I believe I had her support because she saw I was a very good husband and responsible father.   In retrospect, I did not have a lot of conversation about the decision to go overseas with my mom and dad except to let them know I was going. The school and the Dominican Consulate required a letter from someone stating that they would "financially support" me while I was in the Dominican Republic and I typed a letter on behalf of my dad which he signed and I submitted it along with my other documents.

I was advised by Mundial to take a short Spanish language course. I took a six-week evening course at the World Trade Center in New York City that essentially taught the basics, various greetings, salutations, and how to survive day-to-day. There was no focus on the academics or how to have an intellectual conversation, but just enough to get by, which is what I needed. Also, in the interim, I had to figure out a way to come up with the $1,500 semester tuition as well as travel and living costs by September, 1982. In addition, I had to come up with some money to leave Karen to help defray the living expenses at home during my time in the Dominican Republic. Failure was not an option, so during those weeks I turned down no money-making opportunities. I was also still performing life insurance medical exams on the side at all times of the day and night.

At one point, I found myself hoping for some kind of auto accident when I realized I would be several thousand dollars short. Then, guess what happened? Three months before my departure an auto accident actually occurred. I was rear-ended while driving my Dodge Dart in West Orange. After seeing an orthopedic doctor, getting physical therapy, and waiting, I was now able to get the few extra dollars I needed. Talk about Divine Providence and wishful thinking!

Naturally, as I packed to leave for the Dominican Republic, I was filled with some trepidation and second thoughts, but I reenergized myself and I was ready to go. I finished my work assignments at the various venues and thanked everyone for their words of encouragement and letters of recommendation. I also made sure to get all of my employers' contact information. They all gave me open invitations to come back and work with them during the times I would be home on school breaks. I made sure of this by being an excellent worker and always available to cover any and all shifts (days, nights, weekdays, weekends - it did not matter). I left Karen with about $2,500 to cover some of the household expenses and asked her to leave $500 available on the credit card for emergencies. I did not get a personal credit card until I finished medical school in 1986 at the age of 31. Credit cards have ruined more lives, relationships, and marriages than you might imagine.

I arrived in Santo Domingo, Dominican Republic on September 8, 1982 and it was a beautiful day. I exchanged about $50 at the airport. The exchange rate at that time was perhaps 4:1, so I received about 200 pesos. I arrived in the Dominican Republic around 2:00 pm and after getting my luggage, I caught a cab to the Naco region of town where Mundial was located two blocks away. I might add that at this point I had not secured lodging in Santo Domingo prior to my arrival and had planned to stay at Hotel Naco two blocks from the medical school (Mundial) for a couple of days until I found housing. This wasn't good planning on my part, but I was willing to go with the flow. I was a survivor and believed I could handle any situation I'd confront. This was all part of my youthful exuberance, self – assurance, and fearlessness.

In the lobby of Mundial, I met several students who had just arrived or who were already in attendance. It was there that I met Richie (Richworth Philip), who would become my closet friend for the next two years. Richie, originally from Dominica (a small island in the Caribbean) lived in Brooklyn. He was in a similar situation of not having secured housing prior to arrival. As the sun was setting and the evening approaching, Richie and I met a gentleman at the medical school named Juan Polanco who had a home about a mile and a half away which had two adjacent buildings with dormitory-type rooms called la pensione in the back for students. Polanco, as we called him, would often come to the school when a new crop of students arrived each term looking for renters. By sundown, Richie and I were eating dinner at what became known as Casa de la Polanco (House of Polanco) which would be our home for the next four terms (two years) while in the Dominican Republic!

So as not to paint the picture of my departure and arrival into the Dominican Republic as easy and everything going 1-2-3, easy as can be, it was anything other than that. Imagine if you can, going to live and study in a foreign country that you have never lived in before. Imagine having to somehow communicate on a daily basis in a language not your own, having to adjust to a foreign culture, government, and cuisine, and having to adapt to a different climate. In addition to that, I left behind family, close friends, and all of the modern day-to-day accoutrements to which we in "The States" are accustomed. I had a lot to learn and adjust to in a very short period of time.

The pensione was laid out in a very interesting arrangement. There were actually two two-story buildings. Richie and I were the last of the students to arrive and there was only one room left in the main building. I agreed to let Richie take that room and I took a room in the other building. I was the only one in the other building. My room was on the second floor and it looked out over the main court. It measured about 6 ft. x 10 ft. (not very large) and had a ceiling light, a bed, and a desk but no dresser and was reminiscent of the room I lived in for five years on South 15th Street in Newark. As usual, when going into any strange living quarters or hotel, I checked out the building, the hallways, and the bathroom which had a rudimentary shower, toilet, and sink. It was definitely nothing elaborate.

I quickly learned that students and most of the non-private housing did not have hot water for the showers. The water pump ran off of electricity that was intermittently functional since in the third world the electrical grid that supplies electricity is very expensive. The electricity went off most nights and thus I learned to study early because it could get dark at a moment's notice. I also learned to take a shower early or else I might not have any water flow. The temperature, even in the heart of winter, never went below 70° and on most days during the year was in the 90's. Since the Dominican Republic is an island (shared with Haiti), it is surrounded by water and thus with the high temperatures the humidity tends to be very high except in the mountainous regions to the west near Haiti.

The house was maintained by three young ladies. The chief was named Maria. The first obligation of the "maids" was to care for the family of the main house and his family. A Dominican wife relied on the maid for the care of the house, the cooking, the cleaning, and the care of the children. Several of the medical students (mainly those from Nigeria with money) who lived in private apartments hired maids which cost about the equivalent of $100 U.S. dollars a month. The maids lived in the housing complex during the week and would return to their own homes, usually many miles away, on Friday afternoons. Most times they had the weekend off. They were considered to be of the lower class in Dominican society.

The Dominican Republic was and is a very poor country, (but not as poor as Haiti), and definitely functioned under a caste system. The strata level in which a Dominican was born was the level he remained in for life unless he was exceptionally bright and happened to stumble across an opportunity. Also, and more so than in the United States, light skin was definitely the preferred skin color. In all of the businesses, such as banks, and offices the people with the "good jobs" were either white or fair-skinned. The darker skinned people all worked in housekeeping or in the fields performing manual labor.

Maria and the staff prepared our meals and offered to launder our personal clothes for one or two pesos per load. However, their method of laundering dated back to our US standards of the 1940's or 50's with old tin wash tubs and wringers. They dried our clothes on clotheslines in the back of the dormitory. I could not wait to get transportation, such as a bike, so I could take my own clothes to the laundry (lavanderia) which was about five miles away.

Chapter 5

The medical school was located about one and a half to two miles from where we lived and since we had no transportation means yet, Richie and I walked to school each day. In fact, at lunch time each day, if we had no classes scheduled we walked home. Noon in the Dominican Republic is the hottest time of the day and occasionally rather than going back to the dorm, we would stay at the school and maybe get a chimichanga (like a hamburger) across the street at the side walk café.

A day or so after arriving in Santo Domingo, I went to Banco Popular located near the school to start a passbook account. I opened the account with about $500 US and then found the nearest travel agency to purchase my return airline ticket back to New York. Most of the flights to Santo Domingo flew out of either John F. Kennedy or LaGuardia airport. To me, these two tactical moves of purchasing the airline ticket and opening the bank account were very important for security purposes. I wanted to make sure I secured some money at a reputable savings institution and I wanted to ensure I had an airline ticket off the island back home.

I had a duplicate credit card on an account Karen had and I had asked her to keep $500 clear on it in the event I needed it in an emergency. This was not really necessary since I was not taking any chances on her ability to do this and made sure I kept a few dollars in different places in an emergency. I also registered with the US Embassy and made several copies of my passport. I have tried to always live very cautiously, not rely on others, and not to place too much confidence in the foibles of my fellow humans. I was very disciplined back then and the lessons I had learned from "The Nation" (of Islam) really served me well.

I also quickly learned that the law, as we know it in the states, was different in the Dominican Republic. The police in the Dominican Republic had a lot of discretion to make decisions on the spot. If they knew you were American there was some leniency, but that usually came with a small "price" so I always carried some extra pesos with me. I also always carried, at least initially, my small pocket Spanish-English dictionary with me on a daily basis.

As school started, we were given our class schedules (my student number was 82-0232) and the courses we would be taking as first term/first year medical students began. Again, all of the instruction was in English and most of the instructors were Dominican and had spent a fair amount of time in the United States. The first term courses were gross anatomy, embryology, histology, and genetics in addition to a mandatory course in Dominican history and culture. We were all excited and ready to go. Most of us had waited for this opportunity for a long time and as you can imagine were very good students.

I particularly looked forward to gross anatomy and the cadaver lab. I could not wait! Studying anatomy in the Caribbean, to put it mildly, was quite different than in the United States. We had to purchase our own latex gloves and since they were expensive, we would wash them at the end of lab sessions and reuse them over and over until they either tore or the rubber became too brittle. Also, we did not have the best dissecting instruments but we made due with what was available. The air conditioning was not the greatest but was functional and often went out. Our instructor for anatomy lectures was Dr. Francisco Garcia Pereyra. By training, he was a general surgeon and was an excellent instructor.

An instructor I admired deeply was our embryology (fetal development) instructor, Dr. Ulises Perez Placido. This guy was amazing. He had memorized the entire embryology lecture in English and most remarkably would illustrate his drawings on the board using both hands at the same time. This doctor knew his stuff and was a hell of a teacher. In embryology, you systematically study how from the moment of conception each organ system developed over the nine-month gestational period. What was most amazing and a contrast from teachers I had in the United States was that most, if not all of them, taught without notes. This impressed me so much that I have tried to do the same thing when teaching. It can be done if you really know your material and are confident that you know your material.

Histology is the study of normal cells and tissues under a microscope. Our histology instructor had a little more difficult time with English but she did a decent job. In this course, we had to accurately identify all the tissues of the various organs of the body under a microscope and this required knowing the details of the different cells that comprise the heart, liver, brain, smooth muscles, skeletal muscles, etc. Genetics was a little challenging for me since it was one of the courses with which I had no familiarity. Amazingly, I did fairly well in the course with the grade of B.

Overall academically the first term went very well. In anatomy, Richie would come to me for help. Richie, who was better at math, would help me understand and do well in genetics. A fellow student, by the name of Peter, and I were in competition for the best grade in anatomy. Peter, a white guy, could not quite figure out how a black guy could possibly compete with him for an "A," since anatomy lectures and lab exams were fairly difficult. The

African American and Asian students were in support of my winning over Peter and the white students were secretly in support of him. I won by a fraction of a point with a 94 average!

Life outside the classroom, however, was not as easy. I had a history of asthma since early childhood and the humid weather on the island wreaked havoc on my lungs from the first week. In the Dominion Republic, I was able to buy a lot of medications at the pharmacy without a prescription and I knew what asthma meds to purchase. I took the drug Tedral (a drug containing theophylline) just about every day. One of the side effects of Tedral is gastrointestinal upset, namely nausea and diarrhea. I was miserable the entire first term! Wheezing, nausea, and diarrhea was not a good combination for a first-year medical student.

The guys living in the pensione tended to eat meals there. Breakfast (desayuno) was usually very minimal (unlike in the United States), consisting of some type of porridge (which I did not eat) and fruit such as bananas, oranges, and juices as well as occasionally pancakes when the lady of the house was in a good mood. They did not serve bacon, eggs, sausage and the like, at least not to the students. In the Spanish culture, lunch (almuerzo) is a big heavy meal. All lunch meals had rice (arroz) and beans (habichuelas) as well as chicken (pollo) as the main items. In addition, fried or boiled yucca and cassava were also served. Beef was only served about once a week as it was very expensive. With these heavy lunches, you can understand why a siesta (afternoon nap) is usually needed and welcomed! Dinner (cena) was very skimpy and usually without any form of animal protein. Very few of the students got fat unless they had their own apartments, had sponsorship from families, or had money. In addition, walking or riding a bike to class tended to keep us slim and in good shape.

Chapter 6

After an exciting and stimulating first term I took a flight home on December 23, our wedding anniversary day. I had never studied so hard in my life! My focus was keen and based on my grades, I was duly rewarded. I was anxious and could not wait to see Karen and the girls. During the term, we would talk to each other usually on Sunday evenings when the telephone rates were lower, and I knew she would be finished with all of the things she had been doing during the day and relaxed. Also, every week I wrote to her as well as to other members of the family, although not as frequently. After all, most of us had plenty of time to write especially after studying all day. It was a form of stress relief to communicate with someone you knew in a language other than Spanish.

It had been 3 1/2 months since being on American soil and I was ready to go home during winter break and sleep in a real bed, feel cold weather, and take a hot shower if only for a week or so. I had written to my contacts back home about a month before leaving the Dominion Republic making sure the two or three places I had previously worked had some hours for me. I had worked out my budget and if all went well I would make enough to carry me through the next term. I also wanted to purchase a bicycle when I got back to the Dominion Republic so I budgeted for it. The two-mile walks to the school three times a day were getting tedious.

I also had to spend some money at Barnes and Noble bookstore in Manhattan for the textbooks I needed for the second term. This was long before Amazon and the ordering of books and items online. I tried to search for used books whenever possible. Funds were tight but I really did not think about it that much. I knew what I had to do at any cost! I was home for about 10-14 days and worked most of the time. I put in hours at Dr. Darryl Morton's pediatric office and the HIRE facility during the break. Both offices were very gracious in giving me the opportunity to work during my time off. Maintaining these contacts and connections certainly paid off. While other students went home and rested and took "vacation", I worked every shift I could. I also had to spend quality family time with Karen and the girls in the evenings and the two weekends I had off.

As Karen drove me to John F. Kennedy airport in the snow on January 16, 1983, to start the second term, I felt a little better in the sense that at least I knew what to expect. I had made friends at school and we were all now used to living amongst one another. I returned to the Dominican Republic and bought a bike while Richie bought a moped since he had a lot more money. I often got rides with him when we were going somewhere besides the school or on the weekends.

Some of the guys in our circle were Frank Worrell from Alberta, Canada, Emeka Duru, Kenneth Ofoja, John Ogbuneke and Henry from Nigeria. Diane Reynolds was the only black female I knew who was attending Mundial. She was also married and had a strange story which I never quite understood. Others living at the pensione were Don Edwards (from Ohio) and a brother named Mohammad from Egypt who spoke fluent Arabic and Spanish. There were a couple of guys from Thailand and Korea living with us but I do not recall their names. I also learned while I was home during the break that Frank O. had gotten accepted to podiatry school in Harlem, NY and was matriculating there and that another friend from Rutgers, Charles Stephens, was attending Life Chiropractic College in Marietta, GA.

My second term (January to April, 1983) course work consisted of biochemistry, neuroanatomy, epidemiology and community medicine, as well as Intro to Psychiatry. As the term commenced and got into full swing, rumors began circulating regarding the closing of some of the Caribbean medical schools. Several medical schools had cropped up that were started by greedy businessmen seeking to take advantage of a new and growing market of American students. They saw it as a fast way to make money off of unsuspecting students eager to get a medical education. The US Department of Education began investigating this practice and actually closed several schools. As you can imagine, the thought of our school potentially being on the hit list and getting closed down or later losing its accreditation and our diplomas not being worth the paper it was printed on was ever present on all of our minds.

Again, we were fortunate to be at a very small school. Mundial's enrollment was relatively small compared to the others and their administration pretty much followed the rules and guidelines. Richie and I, as well as the others, were on a constant alert and communication with the school's administrators to see if our school was in trouble. We had questioned our decision many a day as to whether we made the right choice of going to the islands to study medicine. Would all of our expenditure of time, money and efforts be a waste? Would we have to return home with nothing to show for our efforts? We just did not know. In the mist of all of this, we still had to study hard and make good grades. I definitely never studied so consistently or hard as I studied while in the Dominican Republic. The pace was fast and left no time for missing classes although several of the students (namely Nigerians) did not take things as seriously. I studied on Saturdays and Sundays usually all day with a break at noon. My method of rewriting all of the class lecture notes helped reinforce the material that was presented in class. This took time but that was the system that worked best for me. Different subjects also required different learning skills.

For example, anatomy required good visual and spatial relationship skills. Biochemistry required learning hundreds of steps in chemical reactions and different branch points to those reactions and what events started and stopped those reactions. Our biochemistry instructor was Maritza de Achecar. She was working towards her PhD and teaching at the same time. She taught from an overhead projector and we marveled at her ability to aptly explain all those biochemical twists and turns and reactions in a way that brought about understanding. I began to see the importance of those general and organic chemistry principles we were mandated to take in undergraduate courses at Rutgers. Another course in the second term was neuroanatomy which is the study of the anatomy of the nervous system. This course was taught by Dr. Juan Santoni. He was one funny dude! Richie and I would make fun of his movements as he taught and tried to illustrate many of the neurological deficits that would occur when disease invaded the nervous system, such as Chorea or St. Vitus Dance. Dr. Santoni was quite the actor as he described an "Egyptian Negress" and marched across the front of the classroom. Neuroanatomy was one tough course. One can only imagine the number of signals, tracts, and pathways running up and down the spinal cord and crisscrossing their way to and from our brain to produce even the slightest movement of our bodies. Truly amazing!

As I was completing the second term of the first year, I realized I had better start thinking about my clinical rotation years (third and fourth years) since none of the Caribbean schools had formal third and fourth clinical years and each student would have to arrange these at hospitals in the United States on their own, and pay for them. The other option was to try to obtain a transfer to a US medical school for the third and fourth years which was a long shot, statistically.

Very few Americans were able to do this especially if they had no connections or did not come from the "right schools" such as long-standing established schools in Guadalajara, Mexico or the schools in Canada. In addition, they would need an exceptional record in medical school, good recommendations, and score in the 90th percentile on the MSKP (Medical Science Knowledge Profile) exam. This exam tested knowledge in the basic sciences taught in the first two years of medical school, namely anatomy, biochemistry, physiology, behavioral science, pathology, Intro to Clinical Diagnosis, and pharmacology. In spite of this, I looked at and studied both options during my 1983 summer vacation back in The States.

I wrote to all of the hospitals I knew of that accepted foreign students for clinical rotations. I looked into transferring back to a US school and saw that the UMDNJ (University of Medicine and Dentistry of New Jersey) accepted about 28 foreign med students each year for transfer out of approximately 500 who applied (roughly 6%). As usual, I was working that summer as a PA at multiple medical offices, mainly in New York and Brooklyn to build up funds for the second year in the Dominican Republic and to help with living expenses at home. I chose to take the MSKP for the first time that summer in mid-June though I had not taken all the courses that are tested on the exam.

Although the MSKP exam is usually taken after the second year, I reasoned I wanted to get an idea of what the exam was like so I sacrificed the dollars and studied like heck in between working and sat for the exam anyway. I am glad that I took the exam when I did because it put me in the mindset of the format and structure of the test and determine the kind of information that would be on the test. I did very well in the areas I had already completed course work in and also in a couple of the other areas, such as pathology and pharmacology which I would not take until the fall and spring terms.

FRANK E. ROBINSON, MD

Chapter 7

I tried to relate the conditions and the daily occurrences in letters and telephone calls to family and friends back home, but I doubt if I was able to accurately describe all that was going on. My fellow students and I managed fairly well in spite of it all. You have to understand that all of us were adventurous and risk takers by nature, evidenced by the very fact that we'd all traveled from other countries to the Dominican Republic. Therefore there was a certain gutsiness in all of us. Premed and medical students are competitive by their very nature, and usually take the most difficult courses and challenge themselves. Most, if not all, of the students (except the Americans) spoke at least two other languages. We knew how to adapt to different environments, people, customs, and cultures and survive and thrive!

To help maintain our sanity, we went to the movies (cine) about twice a month and read the English subtitles so we could understand what was being said. I learned which local barber shop to go to as well as grocery stores (bodegas). We stayed away from the expensive tourist-oriented stores and sites. We journeyed to the beach twice during my entire two-year tour. Both times were in January and both times the temperature was about 72°.

I realized the thought of Karen and the girls being with me in the Dominican Republic during this period of time would have been nice, but it would have not been in any of our best interests. I needed to remain focused. The prevailing conditions under which survival was paramount were crucial. I imagined that dealing with my family and having them adjust to a new culture, a foreign language, and cold water would not have been good. I knew I could deal with the daily inconveniences and uncertainties but I was not sure my wife and two young daughters could or should. To this day I believe, in fact I know, the right decision was made.

I returned to the Dominican Republic in September 1983 ready to kick some butt. The courses would certainly be more interesting and germane to the disease process. The course work consisted of pathology, pharmacology, microbiology, immunology, physiology, physical diagnosis and Intro to Clinical Medicine. We were pretty much used to the routine of living in the islands as our second home. We had made friends and come to accept the laid back, slow-moving ways of this Spanish Caribbean island. My fellow students were more lackadaisical about their future plans than me.

I was absolutely determined to get finished with what I needed to do there and move on.

I understood the system better and resolved in my mind I had to study towards the exam. Whatever the system wanted I was going to give it. For much of my early student career, I believed in learning for learning's sake and getting an understanding of the material and placed getting a grade as a secondary function. While in the Caribbean, I realized it is the grade that matters and the heck with the understanding which could come later. What a revelation!

A troubling event took place in October 1983 and that was on the small Caribbean island of Grenada. About 1,000 American students were attending the medical school there when the United States, under the leadership of President Ronald Reagan, invaded the island. The medical students had to be evacuated and the school temporarily closed. CNN was just becoming a news source and we got most of our news from the television at the local hotels or the newspapers several days after a world event occurred. We lagged several days and sometimes weeks behind things that were happening back home in the United States. On top of that, outside news events were not relevant to our daily lives in the Dominican Republic unless it involved something locally or if it related to US policies and the Dominican medical schools ... then news traveled very fast by word of mouth.

FRANK E. ROBINSON, MD

Chapter 8

The MSKP was an exam required of all foreign medical students seeking transfer to a US medical school after two years abroad. It was the gold standard measurement by which US admissions committees sought to compare the basic science knowledge of students from other countries against US-trained students. The exam covered those areas generally covered in the basic sciences, specifically anatomy, physiology, biochemistry, microbiology, pathology, pharmacology and behavorial science.

Having sat for the MSKP exam the first time one year earlier in the summer of 1983, I approached my fall 1983 studies differently. I had a better idea what the examiners who formatted the test were looking for and their testing style. I was now studying for the test and studying to maximize my MSKP grade to transfer. As I studied, the option of getting a third year clinical clerkship at a hospital was not looking favorable. It would require my traveling to several sites for interviews and even if accepted the tuition for the two years as well as the living costs would be beyond my reach.

I therefore turned my 100% focus to transferring to one of the US schools. In doing my due diligence and research, I reached out to an old friend and former employer, Janice (Jan) Morrell Thomas at Rutgers. I had worked for Jan as a work-study student in the admissions office on the Newark campus in 1974-75. She was in administration and knew a lot of the top people in the Rutgers system throughout the state. It was her calling to aid and assist minority students whenever and however she could. Jan and I have remained friends until this day.

I informed Jan of my current situation in the Dominican Republic and she was surprised and amazed that I had gone overseas to study medicine. I asked her if she knew about the arrangement UMDNJ had in accepting a certain number of foreign medical students into the third-year classes at its Newark and Camden campuses as transfer students. She said she was not aware of this arrangement but would look into it for me. She got back to me later with the news that she knew some of the admissions people at the Camden campus and they informed her of the admission criteria that they used. They required good to excellent MSKP test sores, letters of recommendation, and good grades from the first two years of medical school. She said, unofficially, I had an outside chance of getting in and that she would talk to some people and see what she could do on my behalf.

I recall the ride to John F. Kennedy airport in New York in January, 1984. It was snowing and Karen drove me to the airport and my eldest daughter, Kamilah, was with us. Security at the airport was not as tight as it is today and family or friends could escort a passenger almost to the departure gate. As I was saying goodbye to board the plane, Kamilah started crying. She missed her daddy and did not want to see me go. I am not sure what it was but a tremendous emotion came over me as tears also came into my eyes. I tried to hold the tears back as I kissed her and Karen goodbye and I quickly turned and walked to the airport door. It was at that moment that I said to myself, this is my last flight as a student to the Dominican Republic. Come hell or high water, whatever may be, even if I have to quit medical school, I cannot do this anymore. I truly missed my family and being home! I was going to do whatever it took to get back to the United States permanently. I was not going beyond the second year in the Dominican Republic. I now had more reason than ever before to study my butt off to meet whatever criteria needed to be met to transfer back to the United States. On top of that, money was running out and it would take an Act of Congress to continue. Every dime I had was put into this adventure and I was down to about $1,000 after paying airfare, tuition, books and basic living expenses for the term.

I was able to move a little closer to the school when John Ogbuneke, a Nigerian brother, invited me to share his apartment. My cost was basically the same as I was paying in the pensione at Palanco's and the added features were that John had a maid and color television with cable. At least, I would have a more comfortable living environment for the remaining four months on the island (with air conditioning!!) and would only have to bicycle two blocks to the school. The maid cleaned the apartment and cooked lunch and dinner five days a week. I continued to take my own clothes to the lavanderia.

In the interim, I became aware there were some first-year medical school slots at the UMDNJ Newark campus. In addition to the third-year slot I was seeking, I was encouraged to apply for one of those first-year seats. This would of course translate into me repeating the first two years of medical school but this time in a US school. Also, I was in touch with my old friend Frank O who was finishing the second year at the New York College of Pediatric Medicine in Harlem, NY. Frank put me in touch with Robert (Bob) McDonald who worked in the admissions office at the podiatry school and arranged an interview for me with the head of admissions. I was encouraged and applied for a third year slot at the podiatry school. I had to take the podiatry exam in the spring of 1984 and the exam was similar to the medical school MSKP except there was a strong emphasis on lower extremity (from knee to the foot) anatomy. I scored very well on most of the exam (in the 85-90% percentile) but not so well on the lower extremity part since in medical school there was not a lot of emphasis on that part of the anatomy. In fact, I scored better than most of the second-year podiatry students and I was subsequently offered a third-year slot in the podiatry school in New York.

After completing my final exams in April, 1984, I began making final arrangements to leave the island which had been my home for 16 months. I made sure to get multiple copies of my transcript, both official and unofficial, as well as any last-minute letter of recommendations. Many of my colleagues as well as faculty wished me well in my pursuit to transfer to a US school. I still had to take the MSKP exam in June so my work was still cut out for me. As usual I had stayed in contact with employers so I could hit the ground running and immediately start to work. Specifically, Dr. Wallace Rooney, the Medical Director with Prison Health Services made a part-time slot available for me to fill in for vacationing doctors and PAs. I worked at The Brig in Brooklyn as a PA, mostly the evening shift and on most weekends. I really appreciated the opportunity that was bestowed upon me.

Aunt Carrie had taken ill late in April 1984, several months after an auto accident, and was admitted to Mercer Hospital in Trenton, NJ with a heart condition which did not improve. Regrettably, she passed on April 27, 1984. I am sorry I did not get to see her before her death or be there as moral support for Karen and Uncle John. I was taking final exams so couldn't leave the island immediately. Fortunately, I did get back in time for the funeral in Trenton in early May.

On April 28, 1984, I summoned a taxi which drove me to Las Americas airport in Santo Domingo for the last time. I arrived at the airport early in the morning for the flight to New York. The sun was just rising and it seemed a bit poetic as I stood by the window of the airport. I thought, "Never again will I be looking out this window as a student. I ain't coming back!" I did, however, make myself a promise that one day when we were financially able, Karen and I would return to the Dominican Republic and visit and enjoy all the places I was never able to enjoy while I was there as a student. I vowed to stay at the Hotel Santo Domingo which Richie and I walked by on many occasions marveling about what it must be like to stay in that luxurious hotel on the beach. Needless to say, many years later Karen and I did in fact return to the Dominican Republic and on one of many visits we did stay at that very hotel and enjoyed every bit of it. She even got a chance to visit the site of the pensione in which I lived for three terms as well as meet the Polanco family.

Chapter 9

I made application to UMDNJ both as a first-year and a third-year transfer student. I wanted and needed to cover all bases. In addition, I had the third-year podiatry school seat in my back pocket as insurance. In fact, I actually attended a couple of classes as a third-year podiatry student. A lot was going on at this time. I was like a mouse on a revolving wheel as well as one walking in a maze. I studied daily for the MSKP and waited anxiously for the test scores. I reconnected with Jan and was able to get an interview in Camden for the third-year slot. I was nervous as heck, realizing there was a lot that hung in the balance. I also had to go for an interview in Newark with Dr. Robert Johnson, a black pediatrician, who sat on the admissions committee. He assured me of a greater than 50% chance of getting a first-year seat.

Then something interesting happened. While I was awaiting word from Camden regarding the third-year slot, the Admissions

Chairman at Newark UMDNJ, Dr. Albert Tassoni's office called to officially offer me the first-year slot. In order to accept this offer I would have to withdraw from consideration for the third-year slot in Camden. This was a hell of an ultimatum and a roll of the dice. Was a bird in the hand better than two in the bush? Should I take the guaranteed first-year slot and repeat two years of medical school or should I wait and take a chance on getting the slimmer possibility of a more-coveted third-year slot? I tried to buy some time but Newark gave me a deadline. At the same time, I tried to get Camden to commit or at least show their hand. I called Jan to see if she had any inside information and she had none. She had done all she could do. She had already put in a good word for me and got me in front of the admissions committee. The MSKP scores had just come out and that is what Camden was waiting for to gauge all of the applicants. I had scored decently and still remained in the running. Karen and I talked it over and I chose to take my chances on the third-year slot. I wrote Newark and declined their first-year seat. I then wondered if I had made the wrong decision.

I found out the Camden committee was meeting on a Tuesday afternoon and the decision would come down around 3:00 p.m. I was working at The Brig that day and I could not concentrate. The day seemed like a month as I watched the clock. I had the direct number to the admissions office in Camden and had decided I would call them at 3:15 p.m. sharp. I could feel my heart coming out of my chest and I was getting nauseous as the minutes went by. I nervously dialed the Camden number and it must have rung ten times until someone picked up. I told the person who I was and why I was calling. She put me on hold and came back and it seemed time stood still until she uttered the words, I waited a life time for, "You've been accepted!" I don't believe I heard anything else after that. After catching my breath and thanking every Divine source I could think of, I asked her to repeat her instructions to me. She said I needed to get my final official transcripts to them, pay a $1,500 holding fee and send a letter acknowledging acceptance of the seat. I could not wait to tell Karen but I did not have her office phone number on me. It seemed my whole life changed in one split second. I could not believe it. I had beaten the odds. I was now officially a US medical student. But then I thought, "I don't have $1,500!"

As you can imagine, my acceptance into a US medical school reigns as one of the great achievements in my lifetime and career second only to the medical school graduation day. Little did I know the continued path to the ultimate goal of becoming a full-fledged practicing physician was still many years, miles, heartaches, trials, and tribulations away.

I reflected on the odds I had recently overcome. There had been 500 second-year foreign medical school applicants (200 of whom were from New Jersey) for the 28 available slots in the third year class (5.6%). I was one of the chosen 20 (out of 28) who were from the State of New Jersey. I was the only African American student in the transfer group. All of the remaining students were either Caucasian, Indian, or Asian.

This brings up an interesting point. As I may have alluded to previously. Most, if not all, of my friends who did not gain acceptance into a US med school either gave up trying or went into other ancillary heath fields such as podiatry, optometry, or dentistry (or no medical/health field at all). I was committed and determined to become an MD at all costs. If that meant going overseas, then so be it. I did not want to live a life of regret of, "If I could've, would've, should've." I have always been one to try and give my best even if I did not make it all the way. Henry David Thoreau said, "Some of us live a life of quiet desperation, taking some of our best "stuff" with us to the grave!" I was not going to be one of those people! Being a resident of the State of New Jersey gave each of us, "Jerseyans" a slight advantage since UMDNJ was a state-sponsored academic institution. UMDNJ's medical school system was and still is divided into three campuses: Newark, New Brunswick, and Camden. I had submitted all of the documents the medical school requested and perused the list of additional requested items I had to complete and submit before matriculating at the school in August 1984.

Part of the requirement was that I submit a $1,500 deposit towards matriculation. In addition, we were required as transfer students to take another examination, (the National Medical Board Exam Part One), which is equivalent to the students who were already matriculating at the Camden campus. This examination was quite similar to the MSKP examination we transfer students had just taken and excelled at as part of the transfer process. It was necessary so that on paper all the third year students would be on the same even keel, having taken the same exam.

Again, my dilemma at this point was I was out of cash and wondered where I would get the $1,500 that was required as a deposit. I thought to myself where would I get the money? As a last resort, I called mom and dad and asked them each for $750. Both of them gladly loaned me the money and with that I submitted all of the final documents. After my fellow transfer classmates and I sat for the National Medical Board Part One examination and received passing grades we were ready to start our third-year studies at Rutgers Medical School in Camden, NJ. What a difference it was being a US medical student compared to being a foreign student in the Dominican Republic. The ambience, environment, and respect we were extended was a 180° change from what I had experienced over the prior two years in a foreign medical school.

Epilogue

In this short memoir of "My Dominican Experience", I hope I gave you a glimpse into the life, times, and travails my family and I experienced during one of the first stepping stones in my pursuit of becoming an MD. As I look back, I realize that my years living and studying medicine in the Dominican Republic were some of the most rewarding and educational years academically and personally. It was two years of adventure, risk taking, sacrifice, uncertainty, and tenacity. Above all, it was a statement of true belief in oneself.

These were years that tested my ability to live outside of my comfort zone by living with those from many different cultures and languages as well as adjusting to a different climate with differing social customs. It also demonstrated how, with a willing, hardworking, and loving partner, my wife Karen, I was able to do and accomplish a goal which many believed was impossible. My wife was 99% behind me (I use that figure, since one is never 100%). Even some of those in my own family did not believe it could or should be done.

Along the way, especially during the tough times, many attempted to dissuade me by asking why I would take the chance. They thought it was too uncertain. Many friends said this wild idea of studying medicine overseas is not guaranteed! What if you don't make it? You would have spent all this time, energy, and money for nothing. Why not just settle on being a Physician's Assistant, have a reasonably good life, enjoy yourself, and help raise your family back home? My sense of who I am, *raison d'etre*, as well as my personality, would not allow that.

To me, that would have been a cop out and would have violated my very core and being of self-determination. Everything I had staked my life on was at stake. I knew if I did not at least try, or attempt, I would never be any good to myself, my wife, my children, or my future grandchildren. It was in me to go for the gold and in the end it paid off. Needless to say, at this junction in my career I had no idea what really lay ahead in my pursuit of the coveted MD degree. There were still many meandering roads to travel, endless nights of on-call, never-ending streams of exams to take, and thousands of patients to examine. In spite of it all, I was on a path to *carpe diem*, at all costs! It is my aim and purpose that all those who read this mini tome take from it some of the lessons of life. How when life gives you a lemon you can turn it into lemonade. How even though things may look grim and gloomy and show no possibility of success, that if you keep the faith, work harder than the next guy (or gal), believe in yourself and a power beyond you and within you, that you can do and accomplish just about anything! You must have a goal with a vision, tenacity, and unyielding passion for what you desire most out of life!

In the sequel to "The Dominican Experience" I will continue my autobiography with the story of the long road to attainment of my MD degree. In it, I will lay out the many facets of this journey starting from my completion of medical school studies, then onto my internship and residency years and entering private practice.

I wish you much success and happiness on your life's journey.

You owe it to yourself!

Frank E. Robinson, MD MPH

ABOUT THE AUTHOR

Dr. Frank Robinson is a native of Newark, New Jersey. He completed his undergraduate studies at Rutgers University in New Jersey earning his Bachelors degree. He then went on to matriculate at Long Island University in Brooklyn, New York earning a second Bachelor's degree as a Physician's Assistant. Dr. Robinson proceeded to earn his MD degree at Rutgers Medical School in Camden, NJ and completed a Residency in Family Medicine at Catholic Medical Center in Queens, NY. After finishing his residency, he successfully passed the required exams to become board certified in Family Medicine.

In 1978 he married Karen Collins, who was pursuing graduate level studies in Nursing. After completing his residency, he and his young family, consisting of his wife and 3 children moved to Rocky Mount, North Carolina where he joined a private practice with Dr. James Bryant an older established African American physician. After a short tenure with Dr. James Bryant, Dr. Robinson went into solo private practice.

As one of only a handful of African American physicians in Rocky Mount, Dr. Robinson saw the need for active community involvement to improve the overall care of its citizens. He served on the Board of the American Lung Association and in his last year was the Chairman of the Family Medicine Dept. as well as mentoring Family Medicine Residents at East Carolina School of Medicine in Greenville, NC.

While maintaining a very busy solo practice in Rocky Mount, Dr. Robinson went on to earn his Masters of Public Health degree from The University of North Carolina at Chapel Hill.

After relocating to Georgia in 1993 he opened a solo private practice in Decatur, Ga.; eventually expanding that practice to 3 offices. During this time he became certified as a surgical assistant and assisted a number a surgeons at local hospitals. Dr. Robinson also served as the Medical Director for United Hospice and assisted in developing their initial palliative (end of life) protocols. After developing an interest in Life

Insurance Medicine, Dr. Robinson worked part-time as a Life Insurance and Disability Medical Consultant.

After seven years in private practice in Georgia, Dr. Robinson was offered and accepted a Corporate position in Greensboro, NC as a Vice President Medical Director for Jefferson Pilot Life. He remained in that position for 2 years before answering a burning desire to return to clinical practice. As part of this transition he worked as an Emergency physician as well as a Hospitalist at several hospitals in NC.

Ultimately, he and his wife decided to return to Georgia and Dr. Robinson acknowledging the needs of the under and uninsured decided to take action. He opened a small primary care practice specifically for this group of neglected patients. After 3 years of making a major contribution in this area through this practice, he went into semi-retirement.

Today, Dr. Robinson covers, on a limited basis, several urgent care facilities while also performing dermatologic surgery in Stockbridge , GA. Although he remains highly active in the field of medicine and various business ventures, Dr. Robinson finds time to enjoy writing, reading non-fiction, especially autobiographies, working in his garden and traveling for both relaxation and to attend medical conferences. With no desire to "fully" retire, Dr. Robinson remains involved in community health projects as well as mentoring, doing research and teaching.

APPENDIX

ABOUT THE DOMINICAN REPUBLIC

Source: Wikipedia

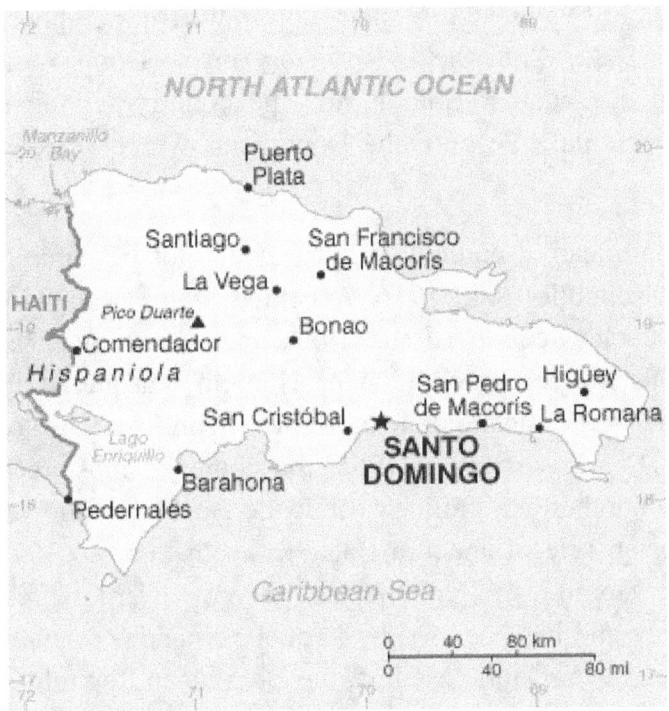

The Dominican Republic (Spanish: República Dominicana [reˈpuβlika ðominiˈkana]) is a sovereign state occupying the eastern five-eighths of the island of Hispaniola, in the Greater Antilles archipelago in the Caribbean region. The western three-eighths of the island is occupied by the nation of Haiti, making Hispaniola one of two Caribbean islands, along with Saint Martin, that are shared by two countries. The Dominican Republic is the second-largest Caribbean nation by area (after Cuba) at 48,445 square kilometers (18,705 sq mi), and third by population with approximately 10 million people, of which approximately three million live in the metropolitan area of Santo Domingo, the capital city.

Christopher Columbus landed on the Western part of Hispaniola, in what is now Haiti, on December 6, 1492. The island became the first seat of Spanish colonial rule in the New World. The Dominican people declared independence in November 1821 but were forcefully annexed by their more powerful neighbor Haiti in February 1822. After the 1844 victory in the Dominican War of Independence against Haitian rule the country fell again under Spanish colonial rule until the Dominican War of Restoration of 1865.

The Dominican Republic experienced mostly internal strife (Second Republic) until 1916. A United States occupation lasted eight years between 1916 and 1924, and a subsequent calm and prosperous six-year period under Horacio Vásquez Lajara was followed by the dictatorship of Rafael Leónidas Trujillo Molina until 1961. A civil war in 1965, the country's most recent, was ended by another U.S. military occupation and was followed by the authoritarian rule of Joaquín Balaguer from 1966 to 1978. Since then, the Dominican Republic has moved toward representative democracy and has been led by Leonel Fernández for most of the time since 1996. Danilo Medina, the Dominican Republic's current president, succeeded Fernandez in 2012, winning 51% of the electoral vote over his opponent, ex-president Hipólito Mejía.

The Dominican Republic has the ninth-largest economy in Latin America and is the largest economy in the Caribbean and Central American region. Though long known for agriculture and mining, the economy is now dominated by services. Over the last two decades, the Dominican Republic have been standing out as one of the fastest-growing economies in the Americas – with an average real GDP growth rate of 5.4% between 1992 and 2014. GDP growth in 2014 and 2015 reached 7.3 and 7.0%, respectively, the highest in the Western Hemisphere. In the first half of 2016 the Dominican economy grew 7.4% continuing its trend of rapid economic growth.

Recent growth has been driven by construction, manufacturing and tourism. Private consumption has been strong, as a result of low inflation (under 1% on average in 2015), job creation, as well as high level of remittances. The Dominican Republic has a stock market, Bolsa de Valores de la Republica Dominicana (BVRD). and advanced telecommunication system and transportation infrastructure. Nevertheless, unemployment, government corruption, and inconsistent electric service remain major problems. The country also has "marked income inequality." International migration affects the Dominican Republic greatly, as it receives and sends large flows of migrants. Mass illegal Haitian immigration and the integration of Dominicans of Haitian descent are major issues. A large Dominican diaspora exists, mostly in the United States, contributes to development, sending billions of dollars to Dominican families in remittances.

The Dominican Republic is the most visited destination in the Caribbean. The year-round golf courses are major attractions. A geographically diverse nation, the Dominican Republic is home to both the Caribbean's tallest mountain peak, Pico Duarte, and the Caribbean's largest lake and point of lowest elevation, Lake Enriquillo. The island has an average temperature of 26 °C (78.8 °F) and great climatic and biological diversity. The country is also the site of the first cathedral, castle, monastery, and fortress built in the Americas, located in Santo Domingo's Colonial Zone, a World Heritage Site. Music and sport are of great importance in the Dominican culture, with Merengue and Bachata as the national dance and music, and baseball as the favorite sport.

PHOTO GALLERY

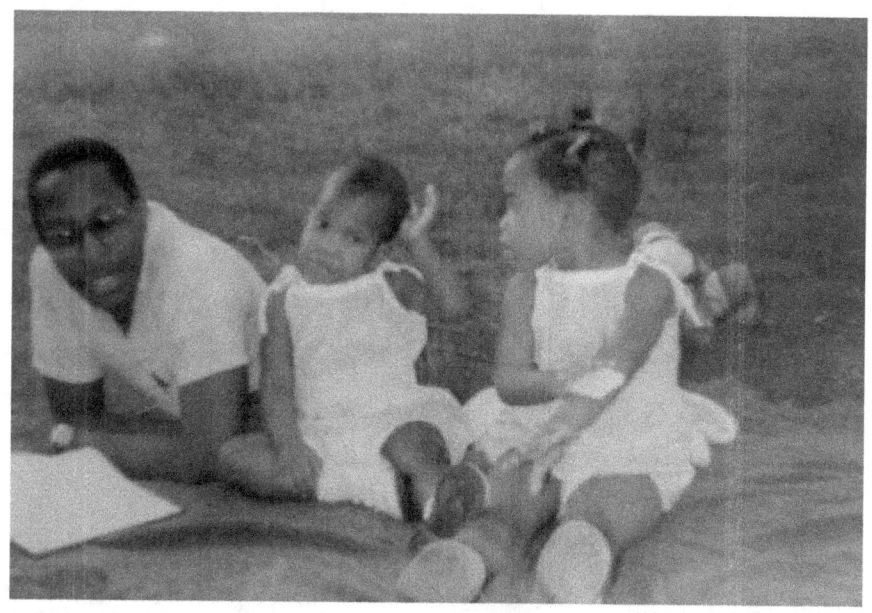

Me with daughters, Aquilah and Kamilah

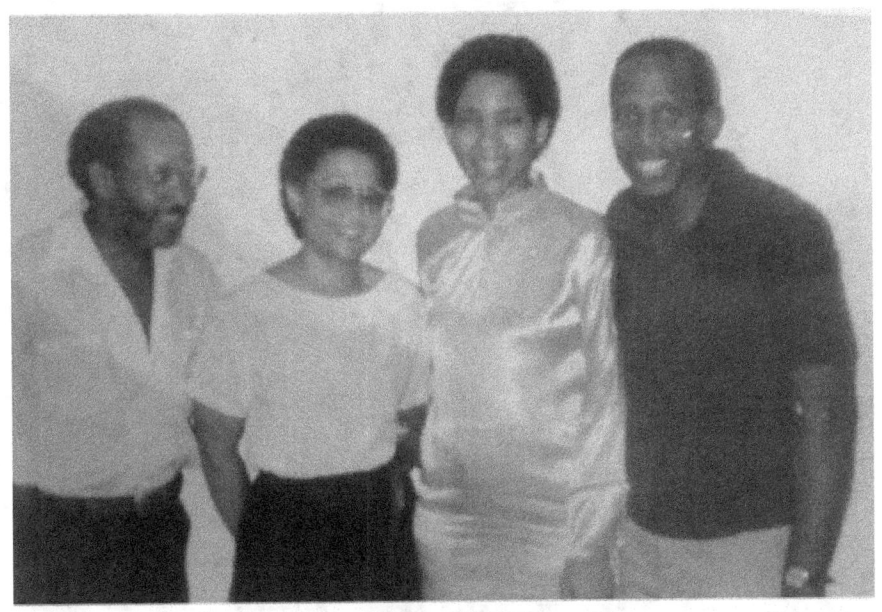

**My friend, Vernon, his lady friend, Karen (wife)
and me - our apartment '82**

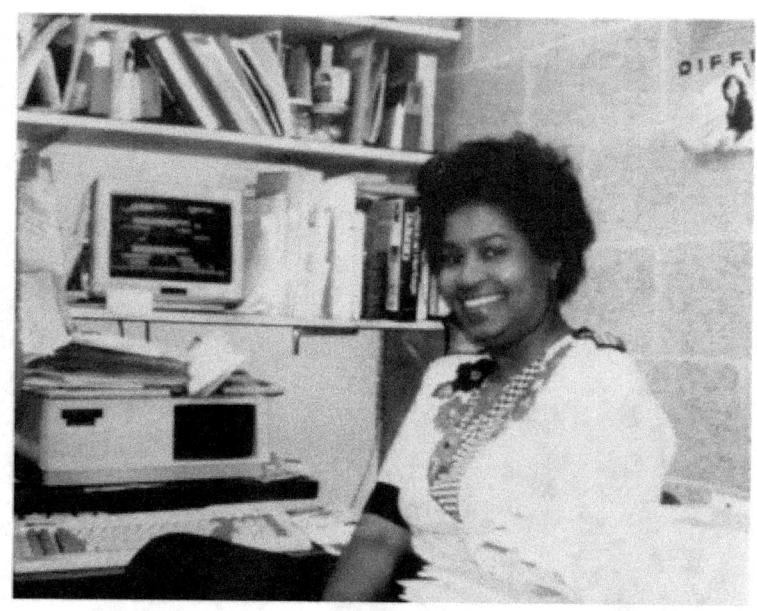

**Ms. Janice Morrell-Thomas
Assisted me in the transfer to UMDNJ-
Rutgers Medical School**

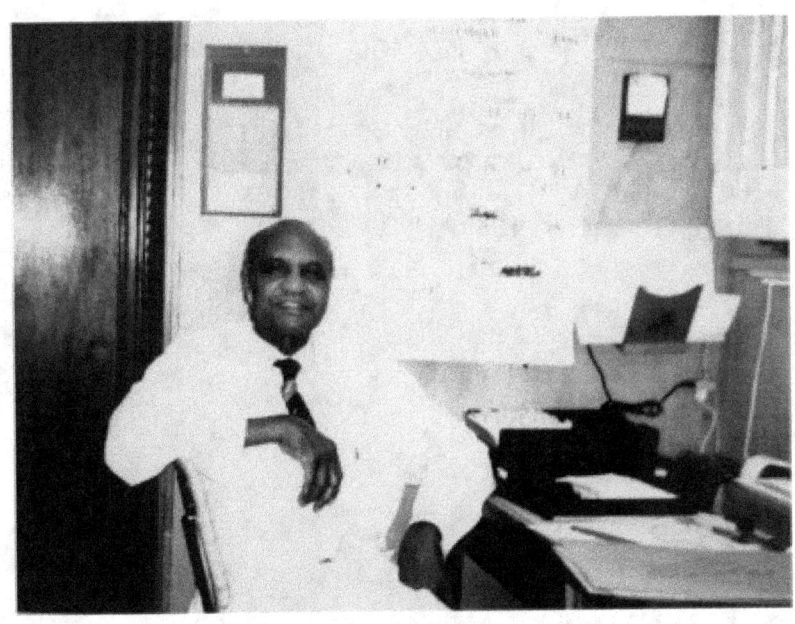

Dr. Edward W. Verner
(Physician Mentor since childhood - Newark, NJ)

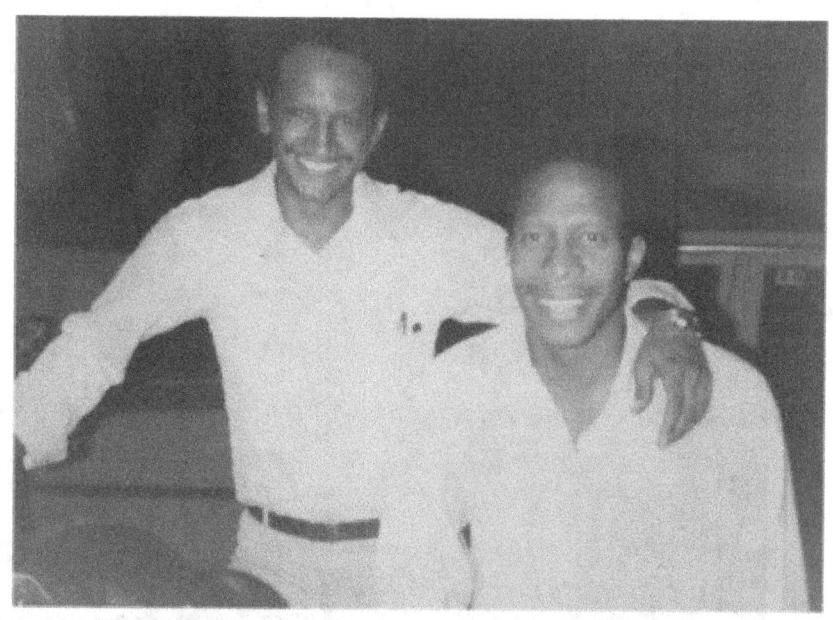

Third year medical student/friend at the Dominican Republic Medical School, Suhait Mohammad (Egypt) and me - 1983

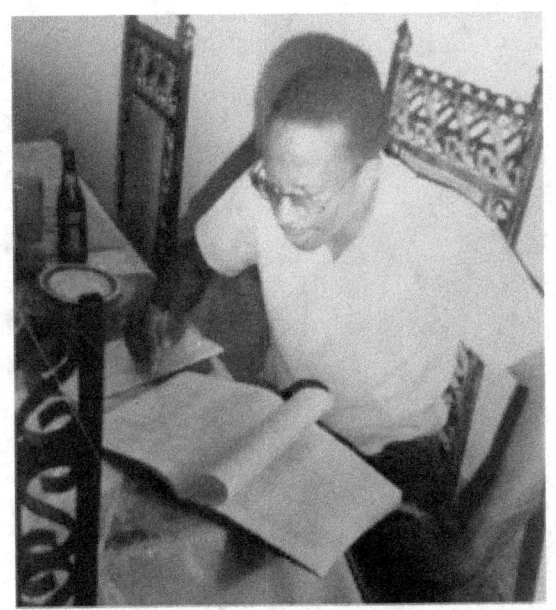

Me, studying in the dining room.

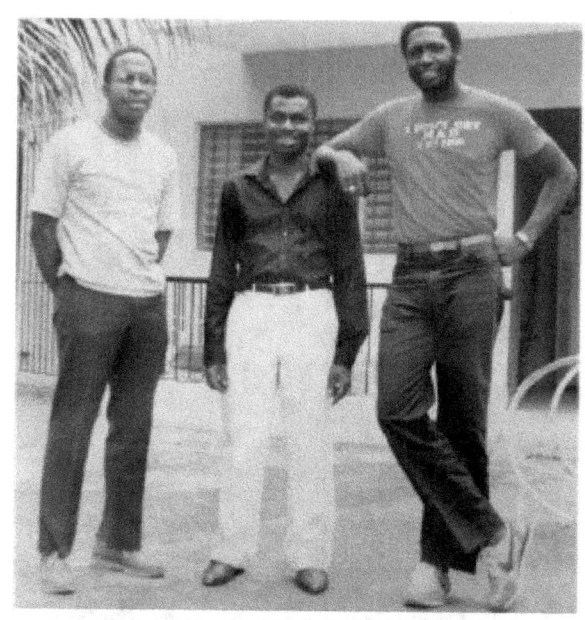

**Emeka Duru, Richie and me
(Outside of my dorm building)**

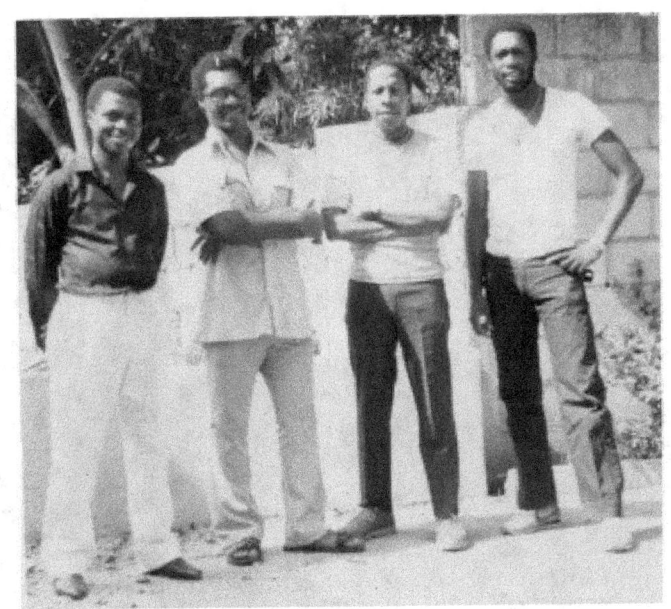

**The Quartet: Emeka Duru, Don
Edwards, Richie Philip and me in the
Pensione Courtyard (1982)**

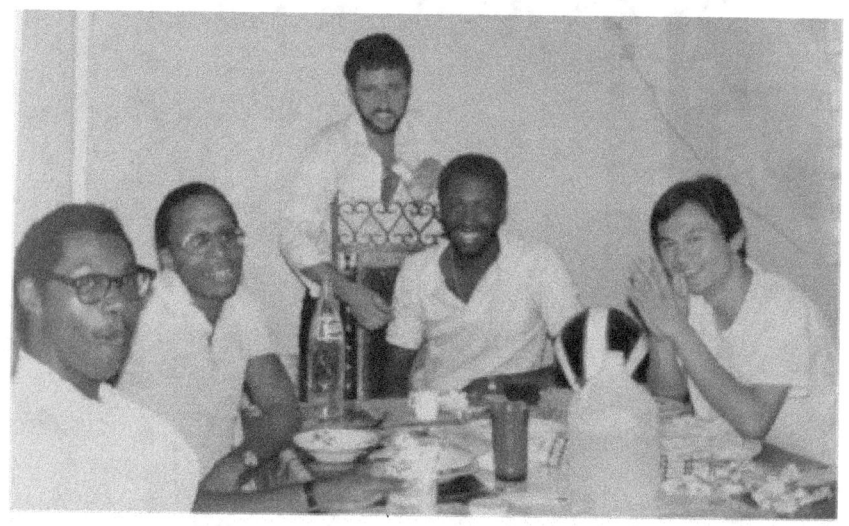

Dining room table at the Pensione (Dorm)

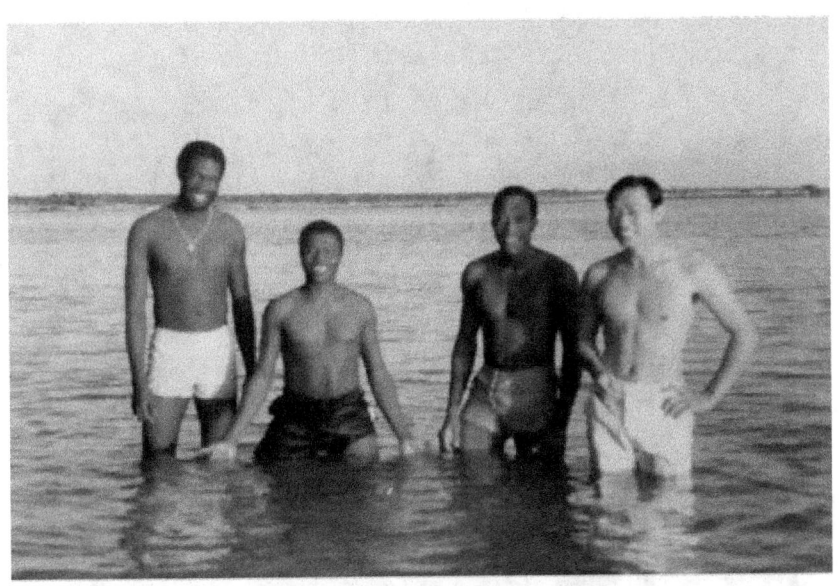

**At the Beach: Richie, Emeka, a
Chinese student and me - January 1983**

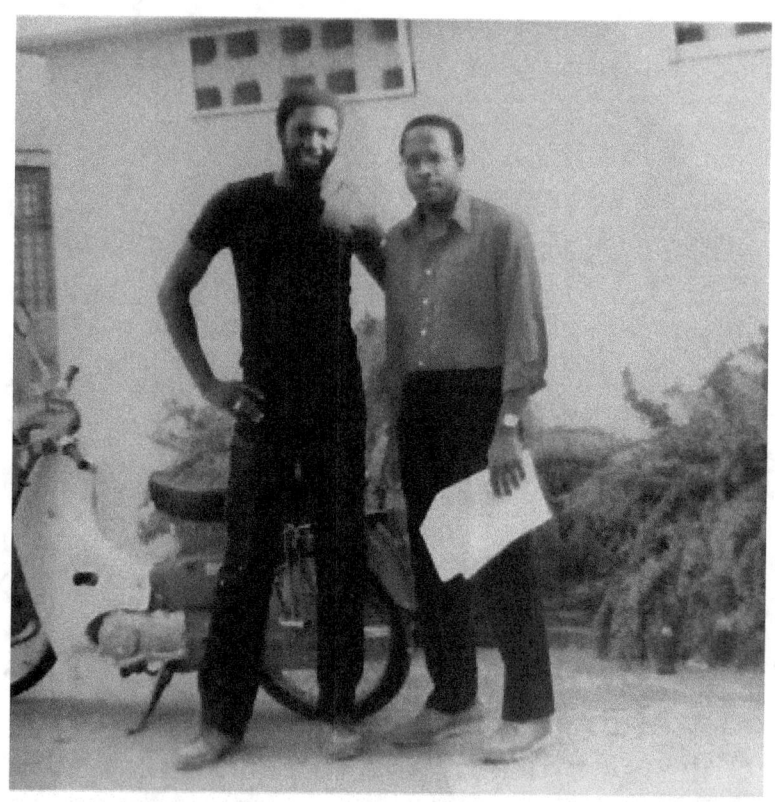

Richie and me by his new Moped

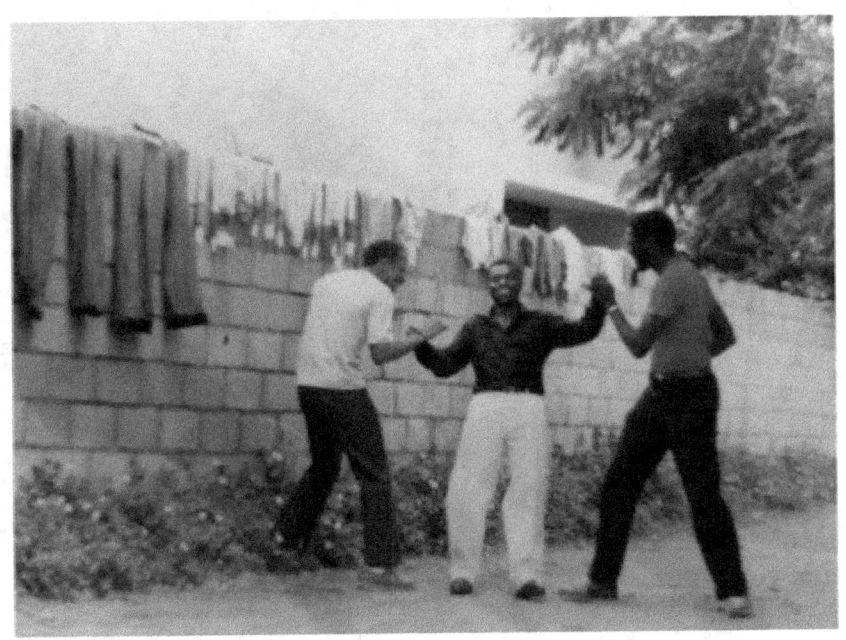

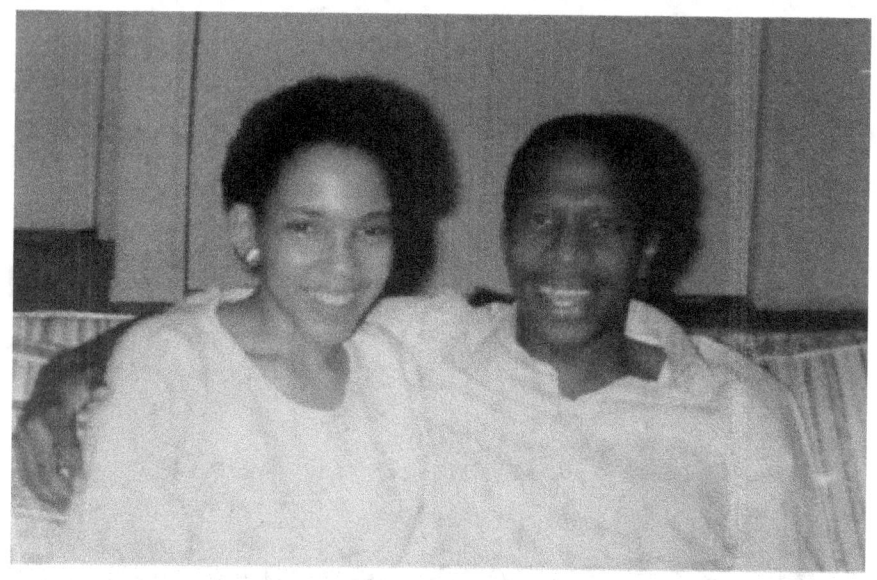

**Karen and I at home in Orange, NJ
During a school break in Summer '83**

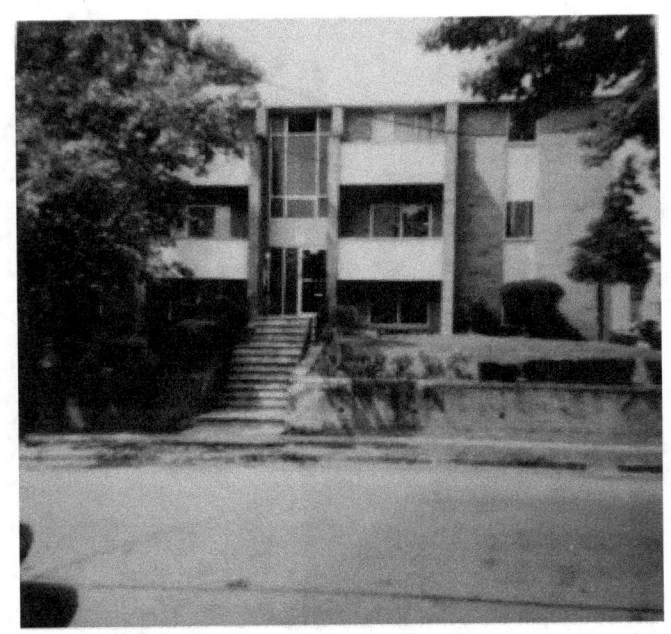

**133 Cleveland St. Orange, NJ
1981-1984**

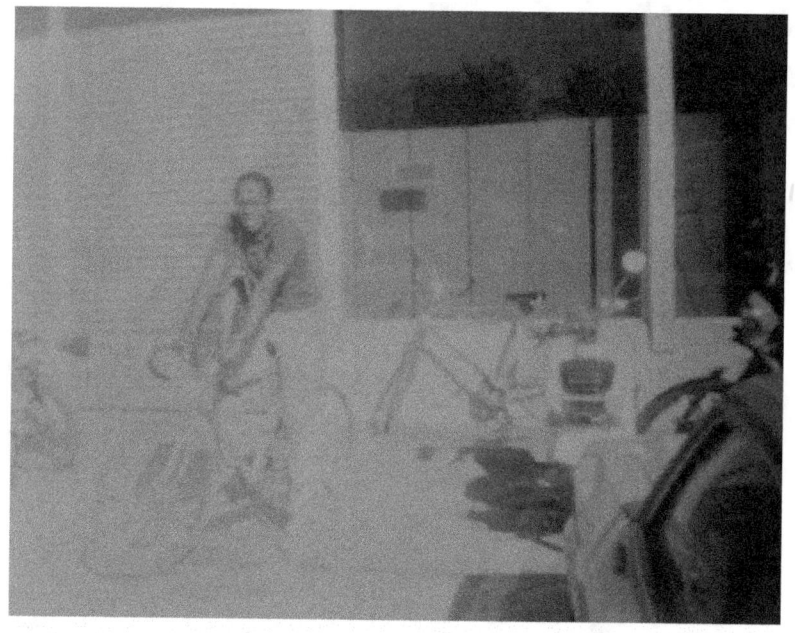

Me on my bike outside the medical school.

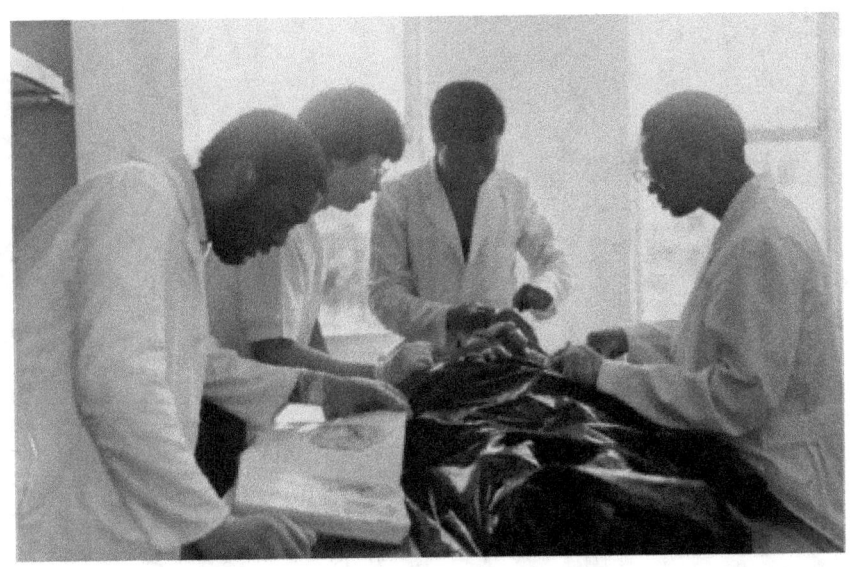

Richie thinking, why is this necessary?

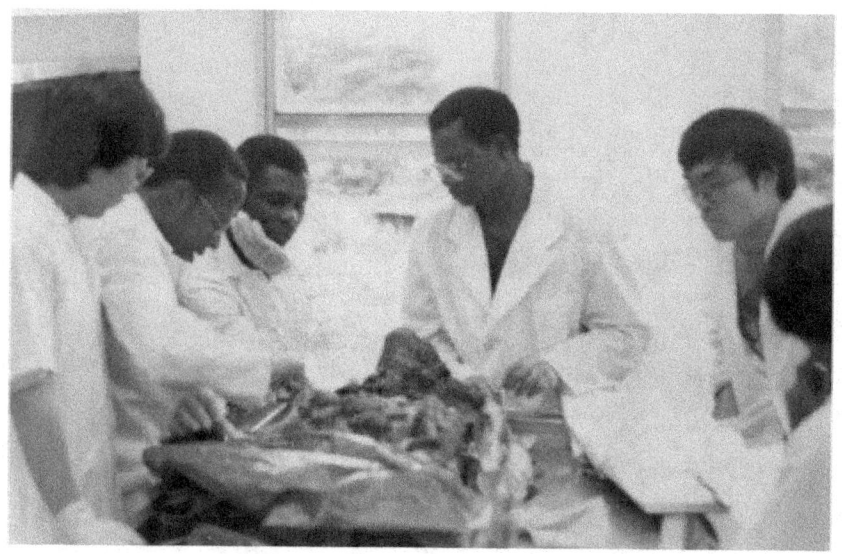

Me at the table; I love Anatomy and dissecting!

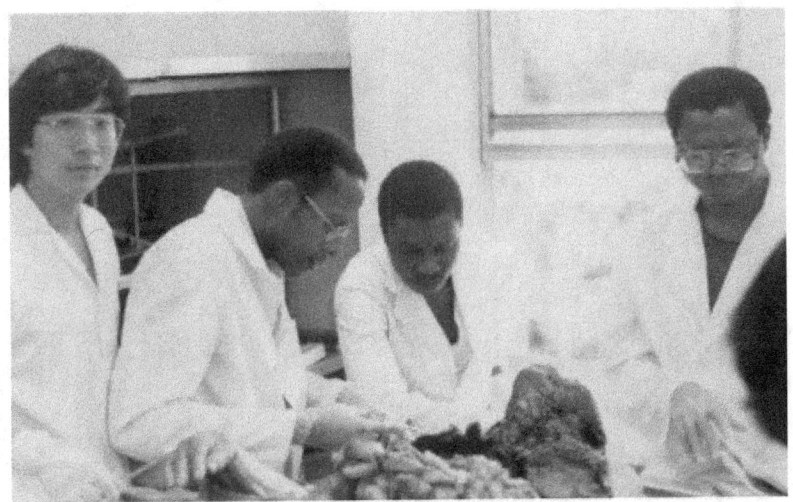

**Emeka, Kenneth and me in Gross Anatomy Lab
Fall 1982 - 1st Semester**

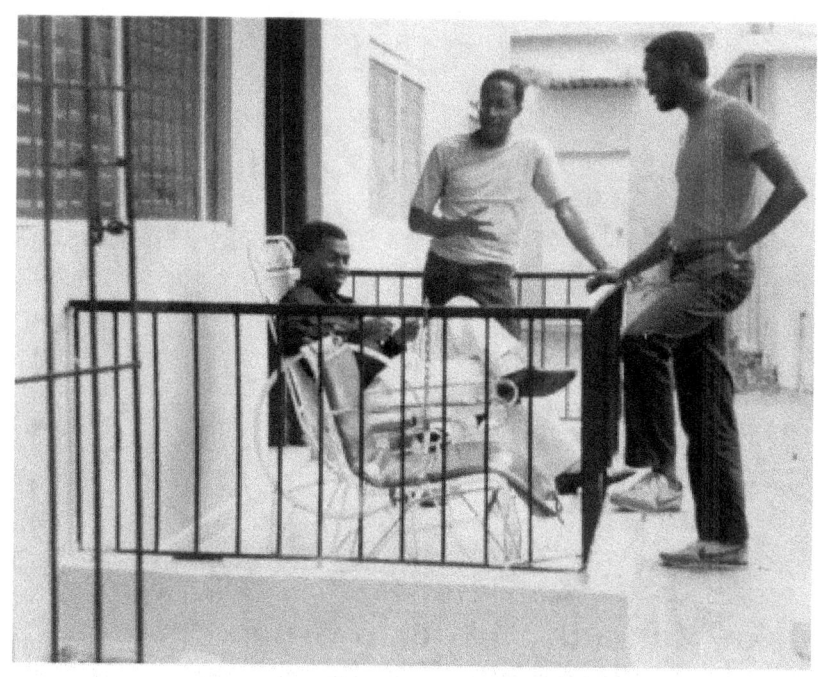

**Me lecturing Emeka (Nigerian) on
American customs.**

FINANCE INFORMATION FOR THE FIRST THREE TRIMESTERS

ESTIMATED EXPENSES

I. TRIMESTER:

Tuition Fee $2,000.00
Application Fee 50.00
Living – Room & Board 1,000.00
Books & Microscope 750.00
*Transportation ....
*Visa Documentation ....

TOTAL FIRST TRIMESTER $3,800.00

II. TRIMESTER:

Tuition Fee $2,000.00
Living – Room & Board 1,000.00
Books 150.00
Miscellaneous 100.00

TOTAL SECOND TRIMESTER 3,250.00

III. TRIMESTER:

Tuition Fee $2,000.00
Living – Room & Board 1,000.00
Books 150.00
Miscellaneous 100.00

TOTAL THIRD TRIMESTER 3,250.00

TOTAL FOR THE FIRST THREE (3) TRIMESTERS .... $10,300.00 **

* Expenses for these items not included

** Amount a little higher to include transportation and visa
documentation expenses.

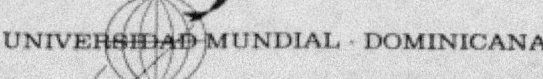

UNIVERSIDAD MUNDIAL · DOMINICANA

FACULTAD DE
CIENCIAS DE LA SALUD   July 28, 1982   ESCUELA DE
                                                                        MEDICINA

Mr. Frank E. Robinson
P. O. Box 331
Irvington, New Jersey 07111

Dear Mr. Robinson:

Confirming our telephone conversation of today, we agreed to transfer your admission to the School of Medicine, World University, Dominican Republic to the September 13, 1982 Trimester, First Trimester level.

Upon acceptance of this notification, you join our Medical School, an academic community committed to the education of physicians of excellence. We are sure that your efforts and dedication will help us in the continuing development of a medical institution deeply aware of its social function.

The tuition fee per trimester is $2,000.00. To confirm your acceptance of this notification it will be necessary that you send us the amount of $1,000.00 which represents half your tuition fee for the trimester, if you would like to have your space reserved. Checks should be made payable to Educational Advancement Fund International, Inc, of World University. There will be a remaining balance of $950.00 which should be paid at the time of registration.

In order to avoid difficulties with the local Immigration Department, we advise that you obtain your Dominican Student visa at the Dominican Consulate nearest your place of residence, upon presentation of this letter of acceptance. Enclosed please find a list of the necessary documents to be presented at the Consulate.

On behalf of the Dean and the Faculty of the School of Medicine, I congratulate you for your achievement in becoming a member of this institution.

Cordially yours,

CARLOS L. LASTRA, Ph. D.
Chairman
Admissions Committee

rpv
Encl.

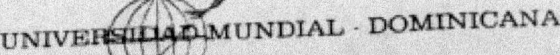

UNIVERSIDAD MUNDIAL · DOMINICANA

FACULTAD DE
CIENCIAS DE LA SALUD

ESCUELA DE
MEDICINA

December 16, 1983

Dear Sir:

This letter is written on behalf of Mr. Frank Robinson, student #82-0232, who is seeking to transfer to your Institution. Mr. Robinson is a student in good standing here at Universidad Mundial Dominicana, School of Medicine.

I have known Mr. Robinson since he began his studies here well over a year ago. During that time, I have had numerous occasions to observe his academic performance including in the Anatomy Course I taught. I can say, at this point, that it is truely a pleasure to write a letter of recommendation for a student like Mr. Robinson. He has done well in all the courses that he has taken.

He is a mature and dedicated student who is well liked by his colleagues and his teachers. I am very confident that Mr. Robinson will perform very well in your School. I, therefore, recommend him for transfer without any reservations.

If you need any additional information, please do not hesitate to contact me.

Sincerely yours,

Francisco García Pereyra, M.D.
Dean, School of Medicine

/mp

LOPE DE VEGA 19, SANTO DOMINGO, ZONA POSTAL No 5
Affiliated with World University, Puerto Rico

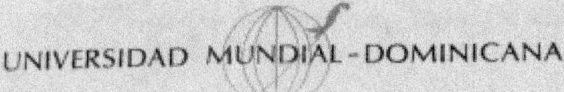

UNIVERSIDAD MUNDIAL - DOMINICANA

FACULTAD DE
CIENCIAS DE LA SALUD

ESCUELA DI
MEDICINA

March 7, 1984

TO WHOM IT MAY CONCERN

This letter is written on behalf of Mr. Frank Robinson,
Student No. WUMS 82-0232, who is seeking clinical clerkships.

Frank was one of my students in the Biochemistry course
I taught during the January-April 1983 term. During this period
of time, Mr. Robinson demonstrated to be a responsible, hard
working student with a great interest in learning the vast implica-
tions of Biochemistry in relationship to the clinical application
of the subject. He is also of a very pleasant disposition and
showed an excellent rapport among colleagues.

I have no hesitation in recommending Mr. Robinson in any
endeavor he decides to undertake. He will achieve his goals as a
result of his dedication and persistence.

Lic. Maritza Penzo de Achecar
Professor and Chairman
Biochemistry Department

MPA:sme

86

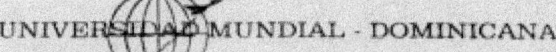

UNIVERSIDAD MUNDIAL - DOMINICANA

FACULTAD DE
CIENCIAS DE LA SALUD

ESCUELA DE
MEDICINA

December 16, 1983

TO WHOM IT MAY CONCERN

This letter of recommendation is written on behalf of
Mr. Frank E. Robinson. I had the pleasure of being his professor
in the freshman Embryology course at the School of Medicine of
Universidad Mundial Dominicana.

Mr. Robinson was one of the best students in his class
and received a grade of A. He impressed me as being a fine and
serious student, eager to learn and hard working.

I have no hesitation in recommending him for any clerkship program at your institution.

Dr. Ulises Perez Placido
Professor of Embryology

EPP:ame

LOPE DE VEGA 19, SANTO DOMINGO, ZONA POSTAL No. 5
Affiliated with World University, Puerto Rico

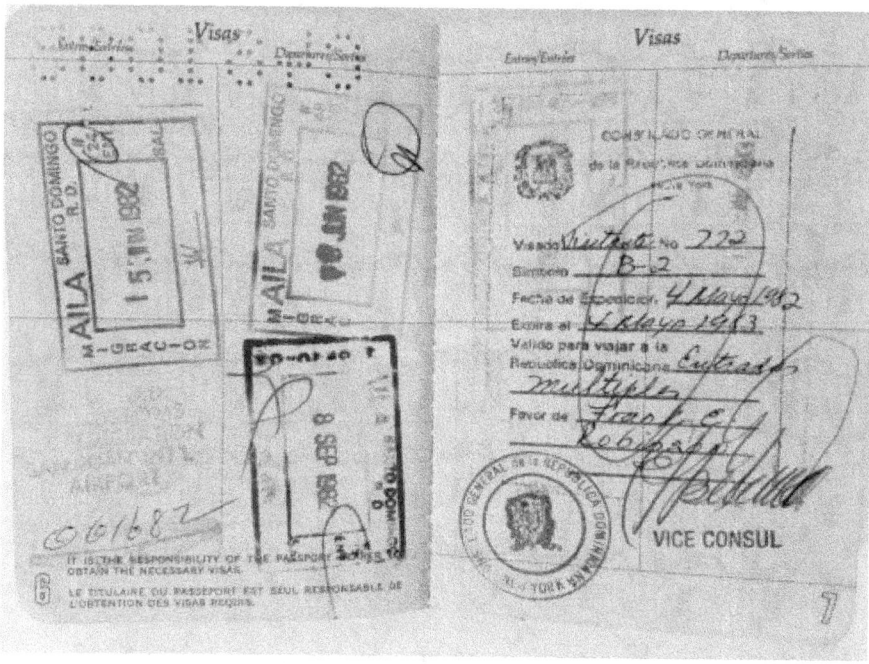

NEWARK STAR LEDGER 10-14-84

Photo by Steve Klaver

28 transfer students admitted by UMDNJ

By JOAN WHITLOW

More than 500 applicants competed to be among the 28 students accepted into the third-year class at the University of Medicine and Dentistry of New Jersey (UMDNJ) Rutgers Medical School this year.

At the monthly meeting of the UMDNJ board, the trustees were told that 24 of the transfer students accepted were New Jersey residents, the bulk of whom spent the first two years of their training at foreign medical schools. More than 200 New Jerseyans, most of them in foreign schools, tried to transfer.

Officials also said the transfers had medical board scores which averaged slightly above the mean for U.S. students and those already enrolled in UMDNJ programs.

Board member Dr. Francis X. Keeley expressed some reservations about the transfer policy and said the school might serve residents better by taking more New Jersey residents into UMDNJ programs as first-year medical students.

The size of medical school classes are governed by accrediting agency approvals.

UMDNJ President Dr. Stanley S. Bergen Jr. said the transfer policy resulted from decisions made in 1979 about filling out the size of the classes going into clinical training at the New Brunswick and Camden health care facilities affiliated with the Rutgers Medical School campuses in Piscataway and Camden.

Bergen agreed with Keeley that on a per-capita basis and in terms of actual numbers, New Jersey has one of the largest contingents of students going out-of-state for a medical education.

That is one of the reasons that many New Jersey residents are attending medical schools in the Caribbean. Most of those schools were organized in recent years to cater to the large numbers of U.S. students who cannot get into medical programs in this country.

The Caribbean schools often lack hospital facilities to provide clinical training in the third and fourth years. Also, because the quality of those foreign schools varies, many graduates are having problems getting licensed and finding postgraduate training programs when they return home.

Keeley said more should be done to keep those students in New Jersey "from day one."

The board was told that some 551 students applied, 212 from New Jersey and 339 out-of-state residents. Also, 199 of the New Jersey applicants were enrolled in foreign schools as were 315 of the out-of-state applicants.

Rutgers Medical School accepts 10 students at its Piscataway campus and 18 at its Camden campus. The UMDNJ's other medical campus, the New Jersey Medical School in Newark, is not taking transfer students.

Twenty-one of the 24 New Jersey residents accepted were attending foreign medical schools, and one of the four out-of-state students transferred from a foreign medical school.

Preference is given to New Jersey residents. The students' undergraduate and medical school records and medical board scores are also used in deciding who gets in.

The mean medical board scores of the newly admitted students was 60.5 compared with 60.4 for those already enrolled and 57.9 from a sampling of U.S. medical schools.

The large number of New Jersey residents in medical schools may be because the state is more affluent than many others and has a large number of doctors, Bergen said.

In addition to the physicians who live and practice in New Jersey, there are others who live here but work in New York or Philadelphia. Historically, the children of physicians make up the single largest contingent among medical students.

NY Amsterdam News 1/22/83

100 PUBLIC NOTICE

Become a Doctor of Metaphysical
Science. Free introductory lectures
every uesday 7 pm—8 pm. at
?aul Robeson Center
50 Greene Ave. Bklyn, NY
(Corner Adelphia St.)
Dr. William Potts, Sr., instructor
636-8269 or 981-5023

GET EASY CREDIT

Delinquent creditors welcomed,
Visa, Master Card Call collect 212-
282-0692

MEDICAL STUDENT
In Need of Financial Assistance.
Please Help, Contact:
Frank E. Robinson
P.O. Box 331
Irvington, N. J. 07111

MY WORLD PRE-SCHOOL
is now enrolling children from
2½ to 5 yrs. old. Don't delay.
Call today 773-5726 or come
to 752 Nostrand Ave. (Bet.
Park & Sterling. Low rates.

PUBLIC ANNOUNCEMENT
Brooklyn Community Board Two is

101 LEGAL N

RECEIVED AT THE OFF
MANAGER, PURCHASI
PLY SERVICES DIV.,
AUTHORITY OF NEW
NEW JERSEY, ONE W(
CENTER, ROOM 74
YORK, N.Y. 10048,
P.M. ON FRIDAY, JA
1983, AT WHICH TIME
SAID PROPOSALS
OPENED AND READ.
CONTRACT DOCUME
OBTAINED AT THE OF
MANAGER, UPON
CONTACT MR. J. D
(212) 466-8219 or (2(
ext. 8219
THE PORT AL
NEW YORK AND

ADVERTISEM
THE PORT AUTH(
NEW YORK AND N
PROPOSAL NC
SEALED PROPOSAL!
REGISTERS WILL BE
THE OFFICE OF TH
PURCHASE AND SUF
DIV., THE PORT A
NEW YORK AND
ONE WORLD TRA
ROOM 74 EAST NE
10048 UNTIL 3:

01-08-84

TO WHOM IT MAY CONCERN

THIS IS TO CERTIFY THAT I RECIEVED THE SUM OF $260.00 ONLY FROM MR. F. ROBINSON FOR HIS JANUARY/FEBUARY RENT AND FOR THE DEPOSIT ON THE TELEPHONE (WHICH IS REFUNDABLE WHEN HIS LEAVING THE APT.)

J. C. Ogbuneke
JOHN C. OGBUNEKE

The A.M.A. Last Week Decided to Crack Down on Fake Degrees and Shoddy Education

Foreign-Trained Doctors In For a Thorough Checkup

NY TIMES   JUNE 29, 84   SEC. 4   P. 24E

By RICHARD D. LYONS

As the social status of doctors has risen — along with their incomes — so has the number of people who try to find a way to profit from that success. In recent years, the medical profession has been worried that its reputation is being undermined by the increasing number of physicians who wear abroad for their training after being rejected by medical schools in the United States. Last week, the American Medical Association ordered the start of what it calls the remedy to the problem — a crackdown on the rise may be the remedy to the problem. In addition, the association said it would cooperate with investigations of fraudulent degrees.

Some changes will take effect almost immediately. Next month's tests given by the Education Commission on Foreign Medical Graduates, for example, will be much more difficult than previous examinations. A foreign graduate seeking a post-graduate position at an American hospital must pass the tests of the commission, which was set up by seven American medical and hospital groups, including the A.M.A. The feeling is, as one A.M.A. official put it at the group's convention in Chicago last week, "[the offshore schools can train their students to pass these new exams, more power to them. The failure rate of students trained abroad is already high. Dr. Samuel Asper of Johns Hopkins University, the commission's chief agent, reported last weekend that of the 19,000 people who entered through medical schools who have shown a record rate in their countries had a percent failed." The examiners demand by places in medical schools

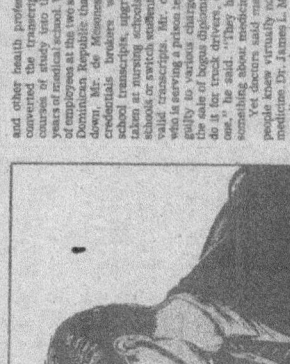

in the United States has led at least 25,000 Americans to enter foreign schools in recent years, enrollments have been rising by 30 percent a year. Above, many medical schools in the world are comparable to those in the United States, most of the American students who go abroad to study medicine go to schools with lower standards. "Money is behind all this," an officer of the A.M.A. said of the proliferation of medical schools in the Caribbean, mainly in the Dominican Republic and Mexico.

Storefront Schools

In some cases, these schools are little more than storefront operations. The Dominican Republic closed two schools in Santo Domingo after it was discovered that they had awarded several thousand fake degrees. Students have tried to use these degrees to enter the hospital residency programs in the United States that would eventually lead to a medical license.

Officials at professional schools abroad say the requirement that foreign medical schools abroad test before they are admitted to American doctors pass a test before they are admitted to American hospital training programs helps block such schemes. But Federal and state investigators have found in the last several years that virtually all tests of medical knowledge have been available for sale, usually after they had been stolen.

Similar investigations are finding that at every point in the educational and licensing system of doctors there is a way around the obstacles. Four years of pre-med studies, for example, can be averted by spending two years in any undergraduate program and then transferring to a medical school in Mexico. Recent disclosures have shown that this is possible at Universidad Noroeste in Tampico and Universidad Valle del Bravo in Reynosa.

Thousands of people have used the services of credentials brokers, who either arrange for acceptance in foreign schools or manufacture the needed documents. One of the biggest scandals in medicine this century involved the fabrication of medical school transcripts through the "upgrading" of courses.

Pedro de Mesones, a Peruvian-born naturalized American, sold-ticted chiropractors, pharmacists, nurses and other health professionals and converted the transcripts of their courses of study into the first two years of medical school. With the help of employees at the two schools in the Dominican Republic that were shut down, Mr. de Mesones and other credentials brokers would forge school transcripts, upgrade courses taken at nursing schools to medical school, or switch students' names in valid transcripts. Mr. de Mesones, who is serving a prison term, pleaded guilty to various charges involving the sale of bogus diplomas. "I didn't do it for truck drivers, or just anybody," he said. "They had to know something about medicine."

Yet doctors said many of these people are virtually nothing about medicine. Dr. Vincent McGuire, former director of medical education at Worcester City Hospital in Worcester, Mass., where several such degree-holders were found working as interns, said most people with training are not well in most circumstances. "But it is the 'zebra', the odd case where the improperly schooled person will most likely fail because he doesn't have the basic scientific knowledge," Dr. McGuire said. "And we can't allow that to happen."

But it has been happening for years because hospitals did not check the credentials of those they hired in foreign schools themselves. Rings of people within the schools themselves fabricated the transcripts but were only hidden them. Dr. Martin H. Desrden founded Credentials Verification International a year ago to deal with the problem. "With someone on the inside," he said, "it is almost impossible to stop such practices."

SUNDAY, JULY 15, 1984   P. 14 Section A(.) NY Times

Dominican Republic Seeks to Restore The Credibility of Its Medical Education

By JOSEPH B. TREASTER
Special to The New York Times

SANTO DOMINGO, Dominican Republic — The Dominican Republic is a country of not quite six million people and a dozen medical schools.

The schools, most of which have been opened in the last 15 years, have attracted thousands of American students and other foreigners who could not get into medical schools elsewhere.

"Some people realized this was a very good business," said Dr. Luis Emilio Montalvo, the president of the recently formed Dominican Council on Higher Education.

He estimated that foreign medical students spent between $40 million and $50 million in the Dominican Republic last year on tuition and living expenses.

Eight weeks ago, the Government closed two of the medical schools on charges that they had been selling diplomas for as much as $50,000 apiece and it has begun investigations into practices at all of the schools.

More May Be Closed

Dr. Montalvo, who has degrees from Fordham University, Loyola University of Chicago and one of the medical schools here, said the investigators had discovered a number of irregularities at the two schools that were closed and that serious questions had been raised about the quality of education at some of the other schools.

"We may have to close three or four more schools," he said in an interview in his steamy office in the Presidential palace, "not because of fraud but because of quality, if we have to close 12 schools, we will do it. We are not going to allow people to deal in higher education as if it were a business."

Most of the medical schools have operated virtually without regulation. Except for the huge state university, which dates to 1538, the schools are privately run.

1,000 Students Left Out

President Salvador Jorge Blanco created the Council on Higher Education with Dr. Montalvo as its head about a year ago, after the arrest and conviction in Alexandria, Va., of a Peruvian-born, naturalized American, Pedro de Mesones, on charges of mail fraud stemming from his fabrication of Dominican diplomas.

The closing of the two schools left more than 1,000 students, mainly Americans, struggling to get transcripts and to find other schools here or elsewhere that will accept them. About 100 who were scheduled to graduate have been unable to get their degrees.

Some critics of the medical schools and of the Government suggest that the schools had not come under closer scrutiny sooner because they were a source of hard currency in a country caught in one of the most severe economic crises in its history.

The income from the Dominican Republic's main export crop, sugar, has fallen while the cost of petroleum and other imports has risen, giving the country a foreign debt of $2.4 billion.

University officials say the fees paid by foreign students have subsidized the educations of tens of thousands of Dominicans. Tuition for foreign medical students ranges from $1,100 to $2,500 a semester; the cost to Dominicans is about $75.

The extent to which individuals have profited from the sale of fraudulent degrees and from the general operation of the medical schools is not clear.

One requirement the Government had imposed on the medical schools was that they deposit the dollar payments of foreign students in the central bank in exchange for pesos at the rate of one peso per dollar. But Dr. Montalvo said he had information that one of the closed medical schools was collecting tuition from 1,300 more students than it had reported to the Government and had apparently been depositing the money somewhere other than in the central bank. The free market rate is nearly three pesos to the dollar.

Schools' Practices Were Known

In numerous recent interviews American students, Dominicans and knowledgeable foreigners said that they had been aware of questionable practices at many of the medical schools for years.

Some of the schools, they said, admit students without high school diplomas. Many do not require college degrees, some give credit for "life experience" and most do not require entering students to take the medical aptitude test that is a prerequisite of medical schools in the United States.

Some American students at the schools spoke highly of the professors and the curriculums. But many said they believed that the education provided by the medical schools here was inferior to that of American schools.

Some students told also of open cheating on examinations. One 30-year-old Canadian student said that before a cardiology examination some students sneaked into the room where the cadavers were kept and ripped out the hearts. The instructor canceled the examination, he said, and went on to other subjects.

"You can pay for anything you want here," said Roger Heil, 26 years old, of Northport, L.I., "diplomas, transcripts, grades, anything."

But Mr. Heil and many other students contended that despite the inadequacies and corruption, by diligent independent study they were able to educate themselves. They said the proof was whether they passed the examinations required of foreign medical students who wish to practice in the United States.

"The grades here don't mean anything to anybody," Mr. Heil said. "If we pass the foreign boards we're doctors. That's what counts."

Many students said that they had heard rumors that diplomas were sold, but that they had said nothing because they did not want to jeopardize their own chances of becoming doctors.

Initially Dominican officials told reporters that they had evidence of the sale of 2,000 medical degrees. But in a recent interview the Attorney General, Américo Espinal Hued, said he did not know how many medical diplomas had been sold.

Dr. Montalvo said that often the process of buying a diploma was spread over a year or two in an attempt to create a history intended to authenticate the false document.

Many "students" never attended classes in the Dominican Republic but paid tuition and eventually went to receive diplomas, Dr. Montalvo said.

The medical credentials of 500 people in New York and of several thousand in California are under investigation, officials in those states have said.

The two medical schools that were closed were the Universidad Centro de Estudios Tecnológicos, usually referred to as Cetec, and Centro de Investigación, Formación y Asistencia Social, or Cifas.

The heads of both schools, who were among 15 Dominicans arrested in connection with the sale of fraudulent diplomas, have denied any wrongdoing.

Students Reminded of Tuition

At the entrance to the four-story office building that houses Cifas, an undated letter taped to the glass door addressed to "all medical students," reads:

"The students that have taken the examination and their tuition are not paid up to date for the semester will have their grades nullified by May 7, 1984. If they pay after this date, they will have to take the make-up examination given from May 20-May 25, 1984. Those students who do not pay by May 20, 1984 will have to repeat the course."

The letter is signed by the rector of Cifas, who identifies herself as Dr. Quisqueya Rivas Jerez. Mrs. Rivas said in an interview that she had a master's degree in sociology from the University of Santo Domingo and an honorary doctorate from the University of San Martin de Porres in Lima, Peru.

Dr. Montalvo said he and others on the Dominican Council of Higher Education are seeking to develop standards for medical schools and a system of accreditation, and are reviewing the credentials of medical instructors. They are also pondering such questions as whether the number of foreign medical students should be restricted and whether medical schools should be permitted to offer programs in English.

"We are very concerned to restore the prestige of our country," Dr. Montalvo said. "If we are going to continue to prepare health resources, we want to guarantee that these resources are of excellent quality."

93

STAR LEDGER
July 22, 1984

ly 22, 1984   Section One; Page 61

READERS' FORUM

Med school, students called victims of bias

DEAR EDITOR:

I am writing to you because of my concern about the education of my fiance who is a student at Ross University School of Medicine in Dominica, West Indies. The school has affiliation agreements with hospitals in New York for the third and fourth years of clinical education of its students, and in New Jersey for fourth year.

The opportunity for my fiance to benefit from the excellent educational programs offered by these hospitals is threatened by actions being taken by the Education Departments of the two states.

In regard to the placement of medical students into clerkship programs, the basic question is whether they are properly prepared for the experience. At the present time New York requires passing of the Medical Sciences Knowledge Profile Examination (MSKP) to qualify for clerkships, and New Jersey will have the same requirement in July of this year. The examination was developed for the use of U.S. medical schools to evaluate applicants for advanced standing admission to include admission into the clinical phase of the educational program. Thus, this examination by itself should be sufficient as a qualifying criterion. If passing MSKP and entering the third year of a New York or New Jersey school qualifies a student for clerkships, why is a Ross student not qualified?

Both states, though, also send teams of consultants to visit the school. In both instances, the teams have developed markedly prejudicial reports which focus not on the educational program but on the ownership of the school.

Ross is privately owned by a businessman who is dedicated to providing the opportunity to study medicine to qualified students who were unable to obtain admission to a U.S. medical school because of the disparity between qualified applicants and available placements. Dr. Ross has devoted his full energies and resources to development of the school into the fine institution it is today.

Please make note of the fact that Ross students have transferred directly into clinical rotations in a number of U.S. medical schools including schools in the states of New York and New Jersey (why are they acceptable as students of U.S. schools but not as students of Ross?)

Also note that both states trust their hospitals to select residents but do not trust them to select clerks. This is most difficult to understand since residents prescribe and treat but medical students don't. Thus we have a situation wherein Ross graduates are accepted to practice medicine in both states while Ross students may be precluded from studying medicine in the same states.

Medical students should be evaluated on their abilities rather than the location or ownership of the school they attend.

Karen Smith,
Livingston

94

EDUCATION

Will offshore medical schools graduate quality physicians?

MILAN KORCOK

Just as medical schools in Canada and the United States face the prospect of cutting enrolments and output of physicians, Charles Modica, chancellor of one of the hemisphere's newest medical schools — and himself a 34-year old medical school reject — adds rooms, faculty, equipment and students to his burgeoning campus in the Caribbean. With health manpower experts predicting that by the year 2000 we will be awash in doctors, Modica encourages his 1000 students at St. George's University School of Medicine on the Spice Island of Grenada to work hard to make it back to the mainland, become licensed and practise what they are convinced is their chosen vocation — medicine. While licensing authorities in Canada and the United States are thinking up new ways to embargo transfer students and graduates from offshore medical schools built for North Americans, Modica leapfrogs from state to state, piloting his own aircraft, lining up hospital clerkships for his students' clinical training.

You could question Modica's timing were it not for the fact that he is winning more than his share of battles and setting licensing authorities in both countries back on the defensive.

Actually, offshore medical schools are not new. The oldest of them all, the Autonomous University of Guadalajara in Mexico, has produced thousands of US and a fair

Milan Korcok is a freelance writer living in Fort Lauderdale Florida

number of Canadian doctors for more than 20 years. Other schools in Italy, in France, in Ireland and other countries have been in the business of taking North American citizens who couldn't gain admittance to American medical schools and training them for MD degrees.

But within the past 5 years, the proliferation of private-profit med-

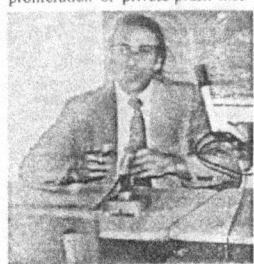

Modica: "Maybe we're cutting a few corners."

ical schools in Mexico, the Dominican Republic, Puerto Rico, and even such tiny Caribbean nations as Dominica, Montserrat, and Grenada, has alarmed licensing authorities; these schools have produced large numbers of students seeking to transfer back into North American schools after their second year abroad, and to receive clinical training in US hospitals. There's alarm because there is no way of making sure that the offshore schools measure up to US and Canadian standards, and there is plenty of evidence that many of them don't

even come close. It's possible to provide books and lecturers and to help students cram through their first two preclinical years; but you can't do clinical training in jungle outposts. It's the lack of this latter component that North American authorities say is the major deficiency of the offshore schools.

To make up for this lack, all offshore schools have given highest priority to getting clinical training programs in mainland hospitals for their students. And no one has been as successful in this endeavour in so short a time as St. George's which now has arrangements with at least 44 hospitals in the United States and six in Britain. To supplement these, there are hospital beds in Grenada and on the neighbouring island of St. Vincent where St. George's has spun off into the affiliated Kingstown Medical College (KMC). KMC is responsible for a fifth semester to prepare students for their clinical training in other countries, and for a ninth semester prior to graduation. It's apparent that the penetration of St. George's graduates into clinical training in so many hospitals is helped along by St. George's practice of donating to the hospital half the tuition fee per student per training semester.

It's a practice Modica has challenged all other schools to meet. He says they haven't so far and probably won't because they are too interested in immediate profits. He says he is willing to wait. "One day I want to be the highest paid chancellor of any medical school in the world", he says. But that will

Medicine

A Crackdown in the Caribbean

Why medical schools are becoming outcasts of the islands

They are situated above grocery stores, in prefab buildings, near noisy bars and open sewers and on the grounds of abandoned convents. Goats and chickens come with the terrain, as do water shortages, blackouts and the occasional political coup. Many lack facilities normally considered standard: research libraries, X-ray machines, fresh cadavers. But for about 15,000 U.S. students desperate to become doctors, the makeshift medical schools that dot the Caribbean represent a last chance. Failure to get into graduate schools in the U.S. once meant flying off to universities in Mexico, Italy or the Philippines. Lately, students have been turning to the Caribbean, where in the past half-dozen years 16 profit-making educational enterprises have flourished on the islands of Montserrat, Antigua, St. Lucia, Dominica, Barbados, St. Vincent, Grenada and the Dominican Republic.

But there is trouble in paradise. Many of the island schools are coming under increasing criticism from U.S. medical authorities for providing inadequate training. Some are suspected of trafficking in phony transcripts. And a number of the medical examinations administered to Caribbean students have been tainted by widespread cheating. Last summer, 9,000 foreign-trained students had to retake tests that allow them to practice in the U.S. because nearly half had seen the questions beforehand. Then in December, U.S. investigators cracked a ring of American and Dominican officials selling bogus diplomas (up to $27,000 for an M.D.). The trail led to two of the Dominican Republic's most successful universities. Last month the schools were closed, their administrators jailed and all student transcripts seized. The action stranded about 900 U.S. students, some of whom were to graduate this year. Cried one American, less than a month from earning her degree: "My life is locked up in there!"

In addition, New York, California and, last week, Florida have imposed strict new requirements on hospitals that accept students from offshore schools. These actions have stirred an emotional debate over how many doctors the country needs and how they are to be trained. Defenders of the offshore schools argue that increasing the supply of physicians will lower medical costs and help deliver health care to places that have long been

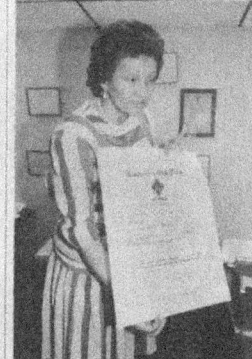

Rector Rivas: "This is no diploma factory!"

underserved: slums, rural areas and state psychiatric hospitals. Critics point out that there is already a doctor glut in many parts of the country and that too often the offshore schools provide second-rate training for third-rate candidates, half of whom fail the U.S. medical qualifying exams each year. "It's a disgrace," says Dr. Vincent Larkin at Brooklyn's Methodist Hospital. "A substantial number don't belong in medical school and will never be able to practice medicine."

A visit to several Caribbean schools offers little that would contradict the arguments of critics. Most operate on shoe-

string budgets and breakneck schedules, cramming a semester's work into four or five weeks. The aptly named Spartan Health Sciences University on St. Lucia has only two full-time professors. The physiology and biochemistry departments occupy one room, separated from the hallway by a beaded rope curtain. The microbiology laboratory consists of a few rough wooden tables. Students are advised to bring their own microscopes.

The Spartan school looks luxurious compared with the St. Lucia School of Medicine, opened with great fanfare last September by Edward Antar, owner of a New York discount electronics chain called Crazy Eddie's. "They had nothing," says Cornelius Lubin, an official in St. Lucia's Ministry of Health. "No labs, no cadavers." The school quietly closed in March. Closed less quietly was the Centro de Investigacion y Formacion Social CIFAS was one of two Dominican medical schools shut down in May as part of the local government's effort to clear the reputation of its university system. Only last April, Rector Quisqueya Rivas Jerez was still insisting that "this is no diploma factory." She has since been arrested and accused of falsifying documents.

Americans are willing to endure much in the hope of becoming physicians. Jeanne O'Connor of Staten Island, N.Y., remembers the day she landed at her school on Montserrat: "Mosquitoes were biting me from all sides. When I got to my dorm there was a tarantula in the closet and a lizard in the bathtub. I sat on my bed and cried." Overcoming these and even greater obstacles, many students attending the better Caribbean schools do manage to emerge with adequate medical educations. Nearly 80% of the students at St. George's University School of Medicine on Grenada passed their qualifying exams last year. The key to their success is the arrangement St. George's has maintained with hospitals across the U.S., by which students spend the last two years of medical school working in wards and gaining practical experience with patients.

Indeed, many hospitals welcome the Caribbean imports. "Our patients are very happy," says Dr. Larkin of Methodist, an inner-city hospital that has trouble attracting U.S. medical students and accepts about 20 offshore transfers every year. Says a nurse from nearby Coney Island Hospital: "The Caribbean students are more humble. The attitude of mainland students is to let others do the dirty work." — *By Philip Elmer-DeWitt. Reported by Marilyn Alva/St. Lucia and Bernard Diederich/Santo Domingo*

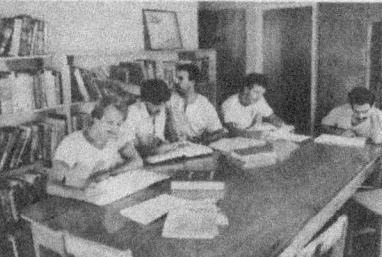

The no-frills medical library of St. Lucia's Spartan University
Students are advised to bring their own microscopes.

www.ingramcontent.com/pod-product-compliance
Lightning Source LLC
Chambersburg PA
CBHW070718210526
45170CB00021B/650

* 9 7 8 1 5 4 6 8 1 4 0 7 8 *